From Blue Ribbon to Code Blue

A Girl's Courage, Her Mother's Love, A Miracle Recovery

JENNIFER MILLER FIELD

WITH

JOANNE FIELD

To Hope + Bob -
Never say Never!
Always keep moving
forward - Never
give up! love! Jennifer

Grove Street Books
Peterborough, New Hampshire
2016

ISBN 978-194193-403-6

Library of Congress Cataloging-in-Publication Data:

Names: Field, Jennifer Miller. | Field, Joanne.
Title: From blue ribbons to code blue : a girl's courage, her mother's love,
a miracle recovery / by Jennifer Miller Field with Joanne Field.
a miracle recovery / by Jennifer Miller Field with Joanne Field.
Description: Peterborough, New Hampshire : Bauhan Publishing, 2016.
Identifiers: LCCN 2015049213 | ISBN 9781941934036 (paperback : alkaline paper)
Subjects: LCSH: Field, Jennifer Miller. | Field, Joanne. | Brain--Wounds and
injuries--Patients--United States--Biography. | Brain--Wounds and
injuries--Patients--Rehabilitation. | Brain--Wounds and
injuries--Patients--Family relationships. | Crash
injuries--Patients--United States--Biography. | Traffic accidents--New
Hampshire. | Horsemen and horsewomen--New Hampshire--Biography. | Teenage
girls--New Hampshire--Biography. | Mothers and daughters--New
Hampshire--Biography.
Classification: LCC RC387.5 .F54 2016 | DDC 617.4/81044092--dc23
LC record available at http://lccn.loc.gov/2015049213

Jennifer Field
J. Field Foundation
P.O. Box 5
White Stone, VA 22578-0005
www.jenniferfield.org

All photographs supplied by the authors.
Painting of "A Distant Memory" on front flap and on page 109 by Jennifer Miller Field
Book design by Kirsty Anderson
Cover design by Henry James
Printed by Versa Press

Grove Street Books
P.O. Box 117
Peterborough, New Hampshire 03458

www.grovestreetbooks.com

Grove Street Books is an imprint of Bauhan Publishing, L.L.C.   Manufactured in the United States of America

From Blue Ribbon to Code Blue

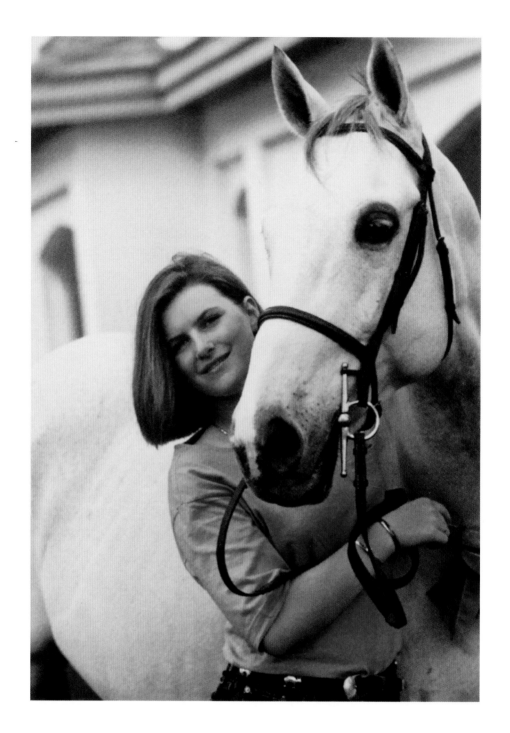

To my mother,
who has given me life not once but twice.
I am here today because of her love, strength, and determination.

CONTENTS

Foreword: *Riding Again*, Alan Weiss, PhD   9

Introduction   11

PART I The Way It Was

Chapter 1 Going for Gold   15
Chapter 2 Stormy Weather   25
Chapter 3 Code Blue   35

PART II The Journey

Chapter 4 The Early Days   43
Chapter 5 The Road to Recovery   53
Chapter 6 Falling Off the Horse   61
Chapter 7 Getting Back on the Horse   67
Chapter 8 Inch by Inch by Inch   70
Chapter 9 A Window to the World   74
Chapter 10 Stalled Out and Restarted   84

PART III A Brave New World

Chapter 11 College Years   90
Chapter 12 My Gramma: A Force of Nature   99
Chapter 13 California (Here I Come)   104
Chapter 14 Creating *A Distant Memory*   111
Chapter 15 The New Normal   118
Chapter 16 Full Circle   125
Chapter 17 Endless Possibilities   129

Joanne's Epilogue   134
Jennifer's Epilogue   136
Acknowledgments   141

Foreword

Riding Again

I was speaking in front of a sold-out auditorium at the Hyatt in Boston, and asked for a volunteer from the hundreds in the seats. As usual, only a dozen people were bold enough to raise their hands, and I noticed the woman with fashion-model good looks smiling in the fourth row. I thought she'd be perfect to join me on stage for a role-play about how to influence a prospect.

As she made her way down the row, she had some difficulty; many may have wondered why people weren't providing a better path. But coming down the aisle it was clear she was having trouble walking. Yet she was deliberate, steadying herself. None of this detracted from her professional appearance—boots, skirt, sweater, hair and makeup done well—and I moved to the stairs to help her ascend.

She took my hand, climbed to the stage, and I helped her onto one of the bar stools, handing her a microphone. I asked her to introduce herself after thanking her for volunteering. That's when the audience realized that she also had some difficulty speaking, a hesitancy that appeared at times.

The large room seemed to be suddenly stopped in time, silent, stunned by this woman who had volunteered, and fascinated (I was told countless times later) by how I would conduct the role-play, which was also being recorded and broadcast.

But I had cheated. I knew this woman. I had been involved in mentoring Jennifer Field for some time. Hundreds of audience members, thousands of viewers, and me on stage weren't about to throw her. She was well on her way to recovery after being thrown by something much worse than anything that could happen on that stage.

As you'll read in the pages ahead, this remarkable woman is recovering from traumatic brain injury as a result of an auto accident. In a nanosecond, she was transformed from a normal young woman into one who needed help to move, to eat, and to think. She could no longer engage in her true love—horseback riding. The extent to which she has engaged in her own rehabilitation, with the intent to help others, is remarkable. But this is so much more than a mere "feel good" story.

Jennifer is an avatar of our humanity. She embodies the power of the human spirit coupled with the pragmatism of leading a productive life. Her message is not just refreshing, but constitutes a reawakening. We recover by helping others to recover. We build our character by helping build the character of others.

A horse didn't throw Jennifer, but circumstances tried to and failed. I'm proud to have been able to work with her, not primarily because I was able to provide some small amount of help, but because I was able to gain so much from her drive, courage, and presence.

It's often said you have to "get back on the horse." But before you can do that, you have to prepare yourself for the race. Read on to prepare yourself for the race of your life.

—Alan Weiss, PhD
November 2015

Introduction

IN 1992 AT THE AGE OF SEVENTEEN, I suffered a traumatic brain injury in a car accident. The doctors didn't expect me to survive, much less thrive. I lay in a coma for two months, unaware of my surroundings. When I eventually awoke I could not walk or talk. I could not open my right eye and I could not swallow. I had a feeding tube inserted in my stomach. One arm had curled upward toward my chest and locked in place. My face showed no expression and I could not even cry. But my long journey to recovery had already begun.

From the day of my accident, family and friends gathered around me to provide love and support. At the center of the group was my mother, who needed that love and support as much as I did. Somehow she summoned the courage to look beyond the dire prognosis for her only child and search out whatever therapies she could find to bring me back. She never gave up believing that I would again live a full and meaningful life—and never let me give up either. This book is our story, and you'll hear both our voices throughout.

My mother said she hated to see me so helpless, because it was so contrary to who she knew I was inside. She was willing to try anything, talk to anyone, and go anywhere no matter how crazy it sounded. I know that willingness helped us in the long run. She refused to listen when the doctors said to her, "Jen will make all of her improvements in the first year, and after that, there will be no more improvement." And they were wrong.

At the one-year anniversary of my accident, I was nowhere close to where I wanted to be, and I realized that my recovery might take a lot more time than we'd all originally thought. Today, twenty-four years later, my brain continues to make improvements. If I haven't seen someone in a while, the first thing that comes out of their mouth is, "Your speech is so much better!" or "Your walking is so much steadier!" or "Your thought process is so much clearer!"

Although I do not believe that there is ever a feeling of complete recovery with a brain injury, the mind and body are constantly changing and creating new pathways with new information. Scientists are now much more aware that the brain has tremendous ability to change its connections based on incoming stimulation.

The brain's plasticity allows it to recover lost function.

My opinion is that you can never think your injury or disease has won. During the early stages of my recovery, I had to find ways of always moving forward. What seemed like small gains ended up being the biggest ones. In the beginning, simply lifting a finger was a victory. I struggled to move from a wheelchair to a cane. I promised myself that when I left the Rehabilitation Institute of Chicago to go home to New Hampshire, I would board the plane using only my own two feet—and that was a promise I did not break.

It still amazes me to look back on how my mom rallied to get me new treatments and therapies she hoped might help me. She considered anything—from live cell injections, to acupuncture (I still remember walking around San Francisco with needles still sticking out of my head!), to neurofeedback, to movement and sound therapies. We quite literally went everywhere—Chicago, Germany, Mexico, Canada, the Bahamas, Connecticut, Washington, D.C., Arizona, New York . . . the list goes on. Once she even considered traveling to consult a healer in Crete. We were lucky that my family had the connections and the means to travel to see these therapists, and even luckier when some of them agreed to come work with me at our home in New Hampshire.

I was very, very lucky to be surrounded by people who believed in the plasticity of the brain and its ability to recover. When I look back at my life since the accident, I feel that most of the therapies I have done and most of the choices I have made were meant to happen. I have invited angels to heal me. I believe in meditation and the spirit world. That is a complete change from the person I was before my accident. But, like so many other parts of me, I've given up my preconceived beliefs from that previous life, because I've learned firsthand that if your heart is in it and you believe, you can will things to work, no matter what they may be.

Today I have regained most of my physical abilities. I graduated from college and live independently. I have written and performed a one-woman show describing my recovery that I have now turned into an inspirational keynote speech. I have also established the J. Field Foundation to support and encourage others who have faced similar physical and mental challenges. I am always so thankful for the many people who come up to me after hearing me speak. I feel lucky to be able to give them more courage to hope and to never give up or give in.

—Jennifer Miller Field
August 2016

Part I

The Way It Was

When I was one, they said I would walk and talk soon—and I did.
When I was ten, they said I would be a champion rider—and I was.
When I was seventeen, they said I would go to the Olympics. . . .

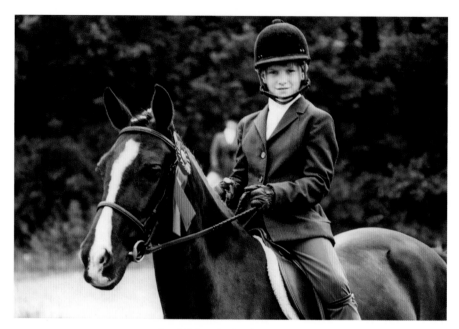

On Midnight Lady, c. 1984

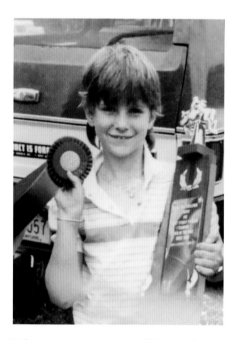

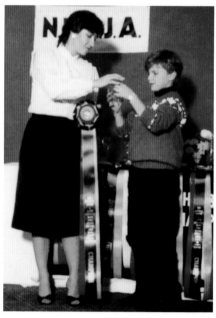

Taking top prize at a small horse show   New Hampshire State Champion, c. 1984

Chapter 1

Going for Gold

I WAS SIX YEARS OLD.

My cousin Marshall was competing in the Junior Jumper division of the South-ampton Horse Show on Long Island, New York. It was early September 1981 and I was as entranced as a six-year-old could be. All I could see was his black velvet hat sailing through the air as he and his horse jumped gracefully over massive fences. Horse and rider were one as they flew over each jump, the horse with his mighty legs tucked underneath him and Marshall perched perfectly over his neck. I could hear the horse's heavy breathing and see the sweat roll down his coat. The beauty of it all fascinated me. At that moment, I knew I wanted this for myself. More than anything, I wanted to be sailing through the air on a strong, beautiful creature. I wanted to reach for the stars.

I remember that day on Long Island so vividly—my remarkable daughter, just six years old, turned to me at her cousin's horse show and said, "Mom, this is what I want to do." I saw how wide Jennifer's eyes were, how determined she was, and I said, "Okay." That was it.

Only weeks after attending that horse show, I was sitting atop Midnight Lady, whom we called Midi. An older pony, Midi might not have been the fanciest mount in the ring, but my trainer thought she would be the right pony to teach me the ins and outs of beginner horse showing.

I loved that pony. I went to Honey Lane Stables every day to clean her stall, groom her, and take lessons. The staff judged us partly on how clean the stalls were, and I remember going so far as to pick up manure with my hands to make sure every inch of the stall was sparkling clean.

Once I had a pony of my own, I surrounded myself with every aspect of horses. Riding became my life. I lived and breathed it. I loved the smell of the barn, and the feel of the powerful animal underneath me.

From the very beginning Jennifer's talent shone. Even at such a young age, she start-ed winning. We began in a kind of "down home" fashion—New Hampshire, where we lived, is very rural, and we were able to participate in 4-H shows and the like.

Midi didn't disappoint. I won my first blue ribbon at a small horse show in New Boston, New Hampshire, when I was eight years old. I had no clue what was going on. We were all novices. My Gramma braided Midi's mane, and I brushed that pony until her coat shone.

Each ribbon won at a show counts for points towards the annual state champi-onship. At the end of the year, Midi and I were crowned state champions of New Hampshire in our division. The ribbon was as big as I was! That feeling of accom-plishment stuck with me. I was obsessed. I wanted more.

We ventured out of state once, to a show in Groton, Massachusetts, where the head of the horse show pulled me aside.

"Listen," she said. "If you give me your daughter, I will make her a champion."

To me, that was a green light. While we didn't end up training with that par-ticular woman, she saw something in my daughter. Jennifer began working with more experienced trainers and we leased a pony called Jet Setter.

When I was ten years old I qualified for the pony finals in Culpepper, Virginia, on my pony Jet Setter. We knew it was a different league, with more than a hundred riders in the whole pony division, and my mom didn't necessarily expect me to place. But I harbored a secret hope: I pictured myself with the blue ribbon. That time, I didn't even come close. I was nowhere near the top eight. Soon after, at my Gramma's urging, we were able to get a fancier pony named Special Effects, whom we called Petey. The next year I returned to Culpepper with Petey and won the championship in the Medium Pony division.

In the fall of 1986, Jennifer was Champion and Grand Champion on Special Effects at the Pennsylvania National Horse Show in Harrisburg, Pennsylvania. When we arrived home to New Hampshire that night, a friend met us at the airport and asked Jen how she did. "Okay," she said in her understated way, and then began handing him trophy after trophy, for a grand total of four.

From that point on, Jennifer started showing in the A-Circuit, which meant she

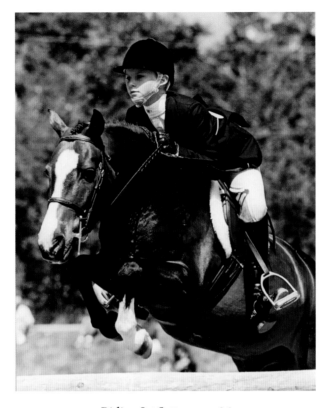

Riding Jet Setter, c. 1986

was competing against the top riders in the country. She loved the high level of competition, and she proved her talent by qualifying each and every year.

I realized very quickly that I was not like all the other kids around me. Focus, drive, and determination overtook me. I had a mission—a mission to be the best I could be, and to walk away from every equestrian competition with a blue ribbon in my hand. I even lost my boyfriend, David, in high school because I could never go to his soccer or lacrosse games. Understandably, he wanted a girlfriend who could be there to cheer him on and offer support, but I was competing in my own sport. I was dedicated to pushing myself and putting in long hours of training for the next competition.

It wasn't just relationships that differed for me—it was childhood and adolescence as a whole. I only went to school Monday through Thursday. Every afternoon

Kristin Connor, childhood best friend

Jen and I met at preschool when we were three years old, riding tricycles and taking naps on mats. We were each other's earliest friends.

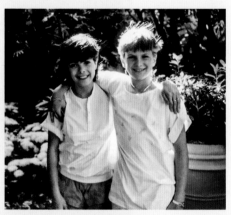

Kristin and Jennifer

Our families helped bond us. Jen had a huge house, stuffed with every toy imaginable, but she loved coming to my house because of my two older brothers who cut her no slack. If they were going to beat me up, they beat her up too!

I knew Jen was well off, but she never flaunted it. She liked getting muddy as we raced each other from one activity to another. We raced scooters and dirt bikes. We jumped on the biggest trampoline you've ever seen. We got into cooking things over and over, like a disgusting mac and cheese recipe we invented. We played constantly in Jen's basement on an indoor swing, challenging each other to see who could swing higher or spin longer.

Once she began riding, I saw that she led kind of a dual life, that included taking limos and going on trips, but she still had to come back to school and to her normal life. Jen was never snobby. She liked living a regular life. She was goofy, happy, and upbeat. As teenagers we attended different high schools and spent less time together; Jen was gone almost every weekend for horse shows. Sometimes I felt Jen was jealous of my freedom. She was kind of on a pedestal as an only child, but I think she just wanted to be like everyone else.

after school I would go home and train for two or three hours. On the weekends I'd compete, or practice for hours if there was no show lined up.

I changed schools . . . a lot. In the winter, I'd go to Florida for three months to ride and, since I wasn't in school for that whole time, I had a tutor. I never participated in school sports or joined after-school clubs, and I didn't have a lot of friends because I wasn't around enough. Some kids were jealous that I was able to leave school so much, but it was just as hard for me to not be a part of the typical school experience. I did, however, have one true, best friend, Kristin, who was everything to me. When I had to be away for riding, she understood . . . and when I returned she was always there for me.

Once I got to high school, I had to make something of a concession. My father, who didn't like my riding very much, wanted me to go to St. Mark's School in Massachusetts. It was a family tradition—he went there, and both my half brother and half sister had gone there too. I knew, though, that I wouldn't be able to ride competitively if I went away to school. So we compromised: I enrolled in a different boarding school close to home—The Dublin School—where I could attend as a day student and keep riding.

Life on the road during horse show season is how I imagine a circus lifestyle might be. We essentially traveled from January to November, participating in shows all over the East Coast. We climbed the equestrian ladder step by step, trading up repeatedly for better horses and more sophisticated trainers as Jennifer got older and better. She was making her mark in that competitive world. She graduated from ponies to horses, participated in equitation (the art of horsemanship and the rider's form), moved on to hunters (which required great skill to maneuver the horse gracefully over each jump), and then on to stadium show jumping.

While Jennifer led a somewhat double life, committed to both school and riding, I led a very solitary one. I was her manager in addition to being her mother—I organized her schedule and drove her to shows and training sessions. It was demanding and expensive to keep going, but it was everything to her—everything to both of us, really—and so it was worth it.

A highlight of my years of intense training was the day I rode into the ring at Madison Square Garden for the Maclay Equitation competition. I was only twelve years old and had no idea what I had gotten myself into. My horse, Double Dare (whom

I called "Dash"), and I were in *far* over our heads, but my trainer at the time, Paul Valier, was very confident in our abilities.

I woke up in the morning excited and ready for the day. I remember thinking in the back of my mind, "Wouldn't it be cool if I actually got a ribbon?" But I quickly put that thought out of my head. There was no way. I knew I was surrounded by amazing horses and riders who were all so much better and more experienced than my horse and I were.

I made sure that morning to do everything I could to prepare my horse and myself. I had memorized the course and went over it and over it in my mind. I imagined Dash and myself sailing smoothly over every jump.

Once the competition began, my focus was as complete as it had been on that day years earlier when I'd watched my cousin Marshall compete: horse and rider were one, horse and rider were everything. My ears were full of the melodic sound of Dash's hooves galloping around the ring, and the swoosh of air as we jumped fence after fence flawlessly. I kept my form all the way around the course. When we finally came to a stop, the crowd erupted in cheers. Paul whooped and whooped. My heart soared with the excitement. I had successfully competed at one of the most prominent horse shows in the United States and taken the Eighth Place ribbon in the Maclay Finals at Madison Square Garden. I was the youngest rider there.

I couldn't believe it. My twelve-year-old daughter was competing at Madison Square Garden, where I had taken her to the circus as a four-year-old. That seemed like only yesterday! I honestly didn't know what to expect. There were 119 other riders, all of them older than Jennifer. I was just so proud that she was competing there.

I had scheduled dinner with some friends for after the competition, and told them I'd call to give them a time once I felt out the day. After I saw how many experienced riders were there, I thought we could probably have an early dinner. But Jennifer made the first cut. Then she made the second cut. Then the third. I kept calling my friends after each round, saying, "I don't know when we will be finished, because she made the next cut!" Eventually she qualified to compete in the top ten. I was so proud and excited.

Jennifer came in eighth that day out of all 120 riders. It was an absolutely thrilling moment for her and for me, the proud mom, her biggest fan. My sister-in-law spoke afterward with one of the judges who said that he had never seen anything like it. In his words, "It was like she had ice water in her veins. I never saw a rider of *her age compete with that kind of resolve. I think she has a great future ahead of her." I realized in that moment that Jennifer had extraordinary talent on a horse. Her trainer and I just stared at each other. We never expected this, but we both knew then that she could go as far as she wanted.*

The world of horses isn't always beautiful. Horses get sick, they go lame. And it's dangerous. Horses are huge, powerful beasts, and even the best riders can't always control them. It was hard sometimes to not be terrified as a mother. I remember sitting in the stands one year in Florida when a horse went completely wild, bucking and bouncing and running all over the place. I wasn't paying it any mind until someone near me said, "Wow, what do you think of Jennifer on that horse?" And I said, "What?" My only consolation was that Jennifer truly did have a way with horses. She was immediately able to control them.

When Jennifer went to the Southampton Horseshow to ride her pony, Jet Setter, I watched as the two of them performed flawlessly until, suddenly, Jet Setter hooked his foot on a fence rail and they went head over heels over the jump. As a mother, it was an awful moment, seeing your daughter spin out of control like that. Before I knew it I was on my feet, headed into the ring, but a man I didn't know pulled me back. "You don't want to go to the other side of that jump," he said. "You don't know what you're going to find."

That kind man went to the other side of the jump for me to see how Jennifer was, and I'm forever grateful. As it turned out, she was lucky and had only hurt her leg, but I took her right home. She was up and riding again before I knew it, but the danger wasn't lost on me.

Some people in the horse world liked to joke that I learned how to ride before I could walk, but I never did that. It was simply that feeling of being one with the horse that kept me dedicated and moving forward. Riding was everything. Not only did I love the horse and the act of riding, I loved the competition. I lived for blue ribbons. I was in love with the adrenaline rush that came with competing, and it made me want to win more than anything.

Over the course of 1991, I progressed to the Grand Prix level of show jumping on my horse Swan Lake, a Selle Français mare that my trainers found for me in France. Swanny was the horse I planned to take to Europe to compete on in the spring. She was the one who helped me make the transition from Junior Jumpers to Grand Prix level, and she was the one, I just knew, who would take me to the Olympics. I

Alison Firestone Robitaille, equestrian friend and competitor

Jen and I rode on the horse show circuit as friends and competitors. Jen was a little older, and I looked up to her. We bonded in part because of our similar dry sense of humor. Jen was serious about riding. She loved her horses. She was very quietly determined. We rooted for each other; we worked with each other despite being competitors.

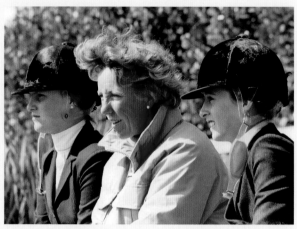

Jennifer, Katie Prudent, and Alison

Our Saturdays started early. We would be in the ring riding our first horse of the day by seven o'clock in the morning. Neither of us were early birds. We would have slept in if we could! We rode four or five horses a day while training. Then we traveled to competitions, which sometimes didn't end until six o'clock in the evening.

Katie Prudent, our trainer, is the best in the business. She was very tough, but in a good way! She pushed us continually to go to the next step. Each morning, we'd walk into the ring and see what Katie had set up for us. We would look at each other, knowing that we were both thinking: "Oh, god! Can we do this?"

It is ironic that Jen's accident did not happen in a ring, where we spent so much time. After her accident, I was not surprised to see Jen progress to where she is now. She was always committed and determined with horses and had respect for them. She transferred that to her recovery. Jen is happy, and that's no surprise either. She was always looking ahead, making everything work, pressing for more.

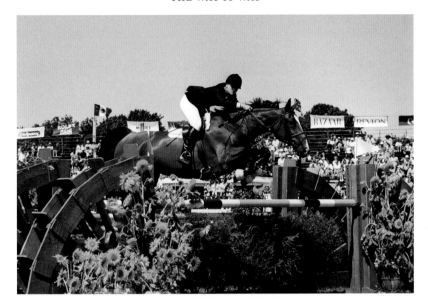

Riding Swan Lake

could envision us clearing each and every fence without hitting a rail. And it wasn't a question of just going to the Olympics as much as being the best I could be there.

After my junior year of high school, I took some summer courses so I could graduate early and go to Europe with my trainers, Katie and Henri Prudent, to compete in some shows over there. I had already been to Biarritz in southern France with them the year before to watch a horseshow, and I couldn't wait to return with Swanny.

I knew that if and when I decided to go to college, I would quit riding for a little while, because I didn't want to divide my time and energy between the two very important worlds. So this was the right time for me to compete in Europe.

The life I was planning for myself included riding at the Olympics every four years and, in between, competing in the best international horse shows I could. By seventeen, I had competed in Canada; in Harrisburg, Pennsylvania; in the Washington International; in Southampton; at the Meadowlands (formerly Madison Square Garden); in Florida; and in California, to name a few places. My childhood dream was coming true.

Katie Prudent, equestrian trainer

Jen was fourteen or fifteen when she began working with me. I assessed her as possessing a lot of talent and a great work ethic. She was determined to be good. I could also tell Joanne was always behind Jen, enabling her to go to shows.

Jen competed at the Medium Junior level with Alison Firestone; they kept each other company. Winners at that level go on to be on the US Olympic Equestrian Team. That is where Alison went, and where I thought Jen would go. I trained Jen to move forward from equitation to the world of jumping horses. As one of the world's top trainers, working with me was incredibly beneficial as well as challenging for Jennifer. But Jen knew that my toughness was all in the service of training. I made Jen want to fight, to win in the horse world.

Training at such a high level demands many hours in the ring, riding many horses a day. Jumping demands not only physical strength, gained through hours and hours of training, it demands courage. Jen wanted to jump big. Though I have trained many students, Jen stood out as a strong athlete and competitor. She later applied that rigor to her recovery.

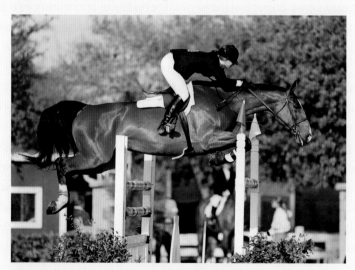

Jumping with Swan Lake

Chapter 2

Stormy Weather

I WANTED TO GO HOME AND CHANGE.

My priority was so simple, so *normal* for a seventeen-year-old girl: I wanted to go home and change my outfit so I would look my best for my new boyfriend, Matt . . . which was why I left school early that November day in 1992, with plans to return and meet Matt there later. My mom was going away for the weekend, and I was excited to think of spending time alone with Matt doing what all seventeen-year-olds want to do—have fun without parental supervision. I knew the weather forecast was for snow, saw the flakes beginning to fall out of the gray sky, but I was determined to go home and get out of my school clothes. With a romantic weekend in mind, I got in my car and began the trip home on the twisting, turning roads of rural New Hampshire. My friend Laura was supposed to be in the car with me, but at the last minute she was called back to give a school tour.

It was November 17, and an early winter storm had begun. Freezing rain and heavy snowflakes hit the windshield with increasing frequency as I drove, but I couldn't have cared less—my complete focus was on which pair of jeans I would wear. My mother was going to New York for the weekend, and I was going to be free. At about two o'clock in the afternoon, I was cruising along with Queen's "Under Pressure" blasting on the radio. I was driving way too fast for the snowy conditions, but all I was thinking about was what lay ahead for Matt and me that weekend.

I have absolutely no recollection now of what happened but I was told that I hit black ice and skidded into an oncoming tractor-trailer. The last thing I remember was the piercing sound of metal on metal. The bumper of the eighteen-wheeler came through the passenger-side window. The impact was so severe that my seat collapsed, my head ricocheted back through the driver's side rear window, and shards of glass speared my head.

Thank god for a volunteer firefighter named Bill Beynon. Bill, who was from a nearby town, was off duty but heard about the accident on his CB radio and raced to the scene. When he arrived, he could see that I wasn't breathing. There was a policeman already there but he hadn't been able to open the car door so he had called

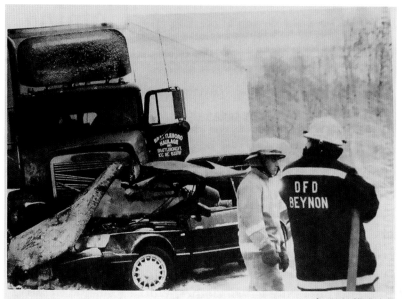

Transcript photo/Mike Cleveland

A 17-year-old Peterborough girl is in critical condition in Concord Hospital, suffering from head injuries in the wake of a crash with a tractor-trailer Tuesday afternoon. According to state police, Jennifer Miller of Sand Hill Road, Peterborough, was heading east on Route 101 in Dublin when she lost control of her 1991 Saab in ice and snow and crossed into the path of the truck, driven by George O'Neill, 31, of Alstead. State police reported that the two collided in T-bone fashion, with the truck striking the passenger side of the Saab. Miller was transported to Monadnock Community Hospital, then transferred to Concord Hospital where she is in the critical care unit.

for the Jaws of Life. Normally, first responders are not supposed to move victims, but Bill knew I wouldn't last long. He ripped open the door and repositioned my head so he could get me breathing again. He broke the rules and did what he had to do—and saved my life.

When I look back on the events of that day, I have to believe that something or someone very powerful was watching over me. There I was at seventeen, trapped inside my crushed car, with an off-duty fireman struggling to help me breathe. When I was born, the doctors had a hard time getting me to breathe; after the accident I felt like I'd been given the gift of life yet again. Months later, when I came out of a coma, I thought about how lucky I was that Bill, a trained fireman, was in the right place at the right time. Now, though, I don't think it was luck. I think it was something more. The eighteenth-century German dramatist and poet Friedrich von Schiller said, "There is no such thing as chance, and what seemed to us merest accident springs from the deepest source of destiny." If that's true, then Bill was meant to be there, to save my life.

Bill Beynon, volunteer firefighter

I was sipping a cup of coffee at a corner store when my phone went off—a car wreck, close by. By the time I got there, the truck driver and a cop were trying to pry the driver's door open. I looked in the car, saw the driver's head twisted so much that I knew it was shutting off her airway; her chest wasn't moving. I thought, *"Man, we gotta get in there!"*

Somehow I got my fingers under the door edge and pulled the door open. Then I turned her head and thought, "We got an airway!" A-B-C, we call it: Airway, Breathing, Circulation. The seat back was broken, and she was lying flat. The EMTs got there and cut the roof off to take her out through the back windshield. In the newspaper picture, you can see my name on the back of my fire jacket.

Jen's was just one of the calls you get emotionally attached to, although you're not supposed to. I felt bad. I remember thinking she was so young and pretty, with her whole life in front of her. I didn't know her from Joe Blow, but I told her later, "I can still remember what you were wearing: a fisherman's knit sweater and a black fuzzy skirt."

While Jen was in the hospital, I used to sneak down on my motorcycle along the road that ran below their barn to ask her horse trainer how she was doing. I did that for the longest time and, you know, the trainer must have told Joanne because one day he said, "You have to stay right here! Joanne wants to meet you."

When Jen finally came home, Joanne invited my girlfriend and me to her homecoming party. She was clumsy, but she could walk by herself. And you had to listen real close to understand what she said, but she could talk. She told me I saved her life, but I didn't do it to be a hero. I did it because it was the right thing to do. It's the way I was raised up. I'd had three years in Vietnam and I was a first responder; my training was: "Get 'em stabilized, bandaged up, and out of there!" I was just doing what I knew had to be done, what I knew how to do.

She tried riding again, to get back to the life she left. But it didn't work out. Vietnam left me with PTSD and Agent Orange stopped me from having kids. I have survivor guilt, too. I was always asking *"Why am I still here?"* It's the same question she asks, *"Why am I still here?"* She's amazing—she totally changed her life—she started all over again.

I was on my way to the airport, but before I boarded my flight, I needed to stop at the veterinarian with my dog, Feather. My friend Mike, the caretaker of my property, was in the car with me. He saw how bad the storm was getting, and he asked me if I thought we should call the school and have someone pick up Jennifer. "No," I said, "maybe this is part of growing up, learning to drive in this weather."

I've replayed that scene in my mind about nine thousand times over the years, and fantasized about turning back the clock to do things differently. I thought I was being a good mother, I thought I was doing the right thing. Later I learned I wouldn't have caught her in time because she left so early. There was nothing I could have done to change things.

Mike and I reached the vet and were in the exam room with my dog when the receptionist came rushing in, saying, "I think you'd better come to the phone, Mrs. Field." I went to the desk, picked up the receiver, and heard a voice say, "Your daughter's been in an accident."

It didn't register at first. She'd been in a small fender bender about three weeks before, and all that had been broken was a little fencepost, so that's what I was thinking. It didn't occur to me that the voice was that of a nurse at Monadnock Community Hospital in Peterborough, until I asked if the accident was bad. When she replied, "You'd better talk to the doctor," I just started screaming.

Barely able to stand, much less talk, I managed to ask the doctor when he came on the line if Jennifer were alive . . . and he said yes. He may have said something else, but I just clung to that answer: "Yes, she's alive. She's being transported to Concord Hospital." I literally dropped everything on the floor and ran for the car. Mike picked up my purse, gathered the dog, and followed me out the door.

My head suffered most of the major trauma, and my brain was starting to swell from the impact of the crash. Time was of the essence. The strength of the storm was increasing so I couldn't be airlifted to Dartmouth Hitchcock, a larger hospital in Hanover, north of where we were. Bleeding heavily and falling deeper and deeper into a coma, I was rushed to the local hospital, Monadnock Community Hospital. In the first of many miracles, this small rural facility had a drug on hand called mannitol, which reduces swelling in the brain. Without it, I might never have made it.

The extent of my injuries was so severe that, after my condition was stable, they decided to send me immediately to the more fully equipped Concord Hospital, nearly an hour away. The blizzard had grounded all methods of air transport, so even though road conditions were clearly treacherous, there was no other choice than to take me by ambulance.

There were no cell phones in 1992. I had a large portable phone that I called "the bag phone" and I remember clutching it to my chest as Mike sped through the storm to the hospital. I was truly in shock. I didn't know who to call or what to do. I just kept repeating, "What do I do, what do I do?—" over and over again. Finally, I came to my senses and remembered John, a friend of my brother's who our family called "The Crisis Buster." He'd know what to do. Luckily I reached him on my first try. He talked me down a bit and offered to call my uncle Robbie, who practiced law in Concord, and ask him to meet us at the emergency room.

I called others on that bag phone. I called Jen's horse trainer, Katie Prudent, who'd had a head injury and knew about some of the neurological teams in the area. I called my mother in Virginia. I didn't reach her then, but she got the message later. When she found out, she moved heaven and earth, and somehow chartered a private plane to fly to the Concord airport . . . in that blizzard!

We got to Concord Hospital before Jennifer. Her ambulance was still on the road from Peterborough. They put me in a tiny room to wait and I nearly went berserk. Uncle Robbie showed up next and tried to comfort me. Finally, I was told that Jennifer had arrived. I ran to the emergency room and there she was on a gurney, looking absolutely perfect—except for the giant clamp on her head that was holding her scalp together.

The doctors explained to me that Jennifer was in a deep coma from the severity of her head injury. They were "bagging her," pumping air into her lungs as they wheeled her in, because she could no longer breathe on her own. I grabbed onto the gurney and wouldn't let go. I remember saying, maybe screaming, over and over again, "Jen, I'm here, and it's going to be okay. Fight, Jennifer, fight!"

At that moment, Carol Connor and her daughter Kristin, Jennifer's best friend, arrived in the emergency room. By some twist of fate, Kristin had been caught in the traffic on Route 101 caused by Jen's accident. When the

Angie Dennis, RN, Concord Hospital

The ER notified us: "Multi-trauma patient coming in, not sure she will make it."
It was a snowy afternoon. I was the first person there, meeting the family—it
was awful—what do you tell them? Jen was pretty broken.

We weren't sure if she'd stay; her family wanted to move her. But Jen was
like broken glass; the amount of head trauma made her too unstable to trans-
fer; she would have died. All day and all night, the family took shifts: Gramma,
Joanne, and Jen's boyfriend, Matt. No one knew if she would make it. It was
sad to see. It was impossible to throw them out. They were such advocates, a
tough group. No flowers are allowed in the ICU, but they brought other favor-
ites to decorate—a clock shaped like a rooster that crowed every hour, lots
of pictures of Jen riding, a scented silk-and-lace pillow. They had little rituals,
and they talked to her about the photos. Joanne and Gramma helped give us
a picture of who Jen really was. They filled us in, so she wasn't just another
broken person, just another patient we were helping.

I used to tell the family, "You can love her, but you sit here. Quietly!" I wanted them to understand the boundaries: you can't keep touching the patient;
it causes harm. You don't want to over stimulate! We monitored Jen's brain
pressure every two hours. And she was on ventilation, so we suctioned her
every two hours, too. Patients can stay in that vegetative state forever. No one
has a crystal ball to predict when or if they will respond.

It was hard to see—Jen drooled a lot, especially when we were turning her.
Her eyes would open, but there was nobody there. Then, after a while, she became a wild child! We put seizure pads on the sides of her bed. She tried to crawl
out of bed. She ripped everything off—her monitors, even her IVs! And she wanted
to be naked—I don't know why! We told the family: these things are normal.

She was in ICU for a month, before she was moved to Pediatrics. The family asked the hospital to allow three RNs to stay with her, to provide continuity
of care since we already had a rapport. Later, after she left Concord Hospital,
I went down to see her at Northeast Rehab a few times. I was amazed at the
care she got and the progress she made. Some patients get forgotten in rehab;
Jen's a miracle recovery.

traffic cleared and she drove by a mangled black Saab, she thought to herself, "There's no way that's Jennifer." Very soon after she was horrified to find out that, in fact, it was.

We were still in the emergency room when my mother arrived. I threw myself into her arms just like a child and sobbed and sobbed and sobbed. I thought that I would never be able to stop. I could not grasp the enormity of what had happened. I felt like my life had fallen apart and would not be worth living if Jennifer could not get better. It was so isolating. I felt like I was in a room with just me and Jennifer, though there were a million other people around. I kept saying, "Fight, Jen, fight! I am here. You're going to be alright." She had to be alright. Finally, the trauma team told me they needed to take her away to operate so they could remove shards of glass from her scalp. I couldn't believe it! How could she go into surgery in her condition? I begged them not to take her, but of course they did.

The hope was that no glass had penetrated her brain, and it turned out that none had. They sent us up to the intensive care unit waiting room. I had never felt this kind of agony. I thought I was going to break into a thousand pieces. When they finally brought Jen to the ICU, I grabbed onto the gurney with one hand, locked eyes with the nurse, and said, "Don't even think about it!" No one was going to separate me from my daughter again! As long as she was there with me, I could keep going.

Over the next twenty-four hours, friends and family arrived. Jennifer's boyfriend Matt; Jen's cousin Wendy; my good friend Bitsy and her husband Sam from New York; John, the "Crisis Buster," and his wife Peggy; Jennifer's dad Edward and his wife Monina, also from New York. My brother Marshall and his wife Jamee from Chicago arrived, along with a prominent neurosurgeon, Dr. Albert Butler, whom they'd brought to consult with the doctors in Concord. We all moved into the waiting room and clung together both emotionally and physically, and began our healing vigil to bring Jennifer back.

Almost everyone from that original group stayed with us off and on for weeks. I drew strength from them, and from the fact that Jennifer was alive. We created our own microcosm. If anyone had to leave—when Matt left to return to college, for instance—we felt as if a part of the whole was being torn away. Jennifer was never left alone; I was always with her, or someone from the group was always at her side.

Mike Martin, the Fields' property caretaker and friend

I had worked as a caretaker for Mrs. Field for three years before Jennifer's accident. I took care of the property and the animals and went to some of the horse shows. As a caretaker, you are involved on a daily basis with all the family members, and I had become very fond of Mrs. Field and Jennifer. I was driving Mrs. Field to the airport, via the vet, when we got the phone call about Jennifer's accident.

Mrs. Field fell apart like I had never seen her. I knew I had to hold it together for both of us as we made our way through the driving snow to the hospital in Concord. It wasn't easy. I had to concentrate on driving while Mrs. Field tried to reach whomever she could on her "bag phone." When we saw a policeman on the side of road, we stopped to ask directions—this was way before GPS and I wasn't sure where to go. When he heard the situation, the policeman gave us a full police escort to the hospital, lights blazing and sirens blaring.

Mrs. Field was shown to a small room to wait for Jennifer's arrival; I tended to the dogs and tried best I could to help with the hospital paperwork. It was unreal and we were all discombobulated. I still remember the fluorescent lights of the hospital, the noise, and the smell. We couldn't believe it was happening. I'm usually very organized, but later that night I drove to the wrong airport to pick up Mrs. Field's mother, a mistake I would otherwise never make.

The relationship between a caretaker and an employer usually evolves over the years as you grow to know each other better. But in this case, it was like traveling eighty miles an hour and throwing the car into reverse. I was smack in the midst of everything. On the one hand, my job was still to take care of the property and the animals. But my new role, which I felt strongly about, was to be there for Mrs. Field and Jennifer and help in any way I could.

There were good days and bad days, of course, and there were challenges on every one. As soon as you won one battle, you'd face another. When Jennifer was in her coma, Mrs. Field and I watched and waited for signs. We somehow felt that if we could keep a routine, hang onto a pattern, we could help Jennifer get better.

Most hospitals have rules that limit visits in the intensive care unit to fifteen minutes every two hours; luckily they made an exception for our situation. The Concord Hospital was gracious enough to let us be in constant proximity to Jennifer. They even let my mother, Matt, Wendy, and me spend the nights in the day surgery room. People show themselves at their best in times of crisis, and I remember laughing, crying, hugging, and reminiscing with family and friends as we all banded together in the small waiting room. I never would have made it without them. I believe that we were able to impart our healing energy and prayers to Jennifer, and in some way helped her to begin her journey back.

"A Distant Memory"

What's my passion
my life and my passion, succumbing
to a distant memory
of life gone by
strength, life, life, strength
a distant memory, passion
sitting atop a powerful animal
I get goose bumps
in the air flying free
the wind blows and brushes me
a distant memory gone with the wind
trying so hard to be someone
a distant memory free from my life
anger, getting chills
an empty room tears stream down my face
in red, ochre, brown, green and black, life's brushstrokes
creating a masterpiece
movement, power captured within
flying free of a wooden frame and escaping the confines of myself
no boundaries, free
the sound overtaking me
a distant memory, please come back
further and further, a mask awaits
the snow falls
a white palace

—Jennifer

Chapter 3

Code Blue

We developed a routine in the hospital that became our daily life. It was mostly about watching and waiting. My mother would answer all the phone calls that came in because after I said, "Hello," I would just burst into tears, unable to stop crying. She also greeted the many visitors who came by to offer their condolences, and to see Jennifer. I felt I was there to protect Jennifer and that she would not want everybody to see her incapacitated, with all of those tubes coming out of her. I let very few people back to her room. Maybe I didn't want to face up to their comments or engage in a conversation about Jennifer's condition—for me that could make the situation agonizingly real. No one could focus enough to watch television or read a book. Waiting and holding ourselves together became a full-time job. Periodically, our routine would be threatened by changes in Jennifer's condition. One morning at about five o'clock, I was lying on my little cot in the waiting room when I heard a voice over the loudspeaker calling, "Code Blue. Code Blue." The doctors had been trying to re-intubate Jennifer, and I just knew the code was for her. I ran to intensive care and saw her room packed with nurses and doctors. I asked one of the doctors near the back what was happening. "There are too many people," he said, and walked away.

I wanted to kill him, but I went back to my cot and sat huddled in a ball. I couldn't believe he wouldn't find out something for me. I was shaking and praying. This could not be the moment I lost her. Finally, someone came to report that yes, she had stopped breathing, but was stable now. They wanted to bring in an anesthesiologist to complete the intubation. I asked that they call the anesthesiologist who was on duty the night she came in. I figured if he could bring her through that, he could bring her through anything. And he did.

There were other incidents like that that almost pushed me over the edge. But Jennifer pulled through each time, and each time I managed to hold myself together. As the days wore on I just wouldn't acknowledge the possibility that Jen might not survive. I refused to let any of the dire information from the doctors really register. I felt like I was teetering on a tightrope both emotionally and phys-

ically—swaying this way and that, barely balancing—and at some moment, somebody might say the thing I couldn't hear, and I'd fall.

I had to keep myself on that tightrope no matter what. The neurosurgeons held no hope for her recovery, although they never actually said it. But I couldn't allow myself to think that she wouldn't get better. She had to get better. She had to get better or I felt I couldn't go on living. It was almost a selfish thing, but she had to. So I just had to wait. And while I sat by her bedside, I kept picturing her damaged brain and how to fix it. I pictured downed phone lines or an old-fashioned switch-board with the connections ripped out. I concluded that I had to find the therapies that would reconnect her brain.

My diagnosis was a "diffuse closed head injury," which, simply put, means the brain was damaged all over. Although the truck hit on the right side of my car, the whiplash was so severe that the left side of my brain received the greatest trauma. Because the body works in diagonals—the left part of the brain controls the right side of the body, and vice versa—when I eventually awoke, my right side was completely paralyzed. I couldn't walk, talk, or use my right arm, and my right eye was completely closed.

There was a time when my neurosurgeons didn't know if I would survive. I stayed in a coma for two months, I had an antenna that monitored the pressure in my brain jutting out of my head for a week, and my CAT scans showed damage in a multitude of places. I later learned that the night I arrived at the hospital I was submerged in a tub full of ice to try and bring down the swelling in my brain. When doctors tried to insert a permanent breathing tube, they accidentally punctured my lung so they had to put in a second tube to re-inflate it. As my coma progressed, my left arm and leg constantly moved involuntarily, and my right arm curled up to my bicep and locked in position as if set in cement. No one could move it down without fear of breaking it.

The doctors became increasingly worried that Jen would develop "foot drop," a condition in which the feet turn downward like a ballerina's on pointe; it can later inhibit the ability to walk. The doctors wanted to put Jen in casts to keep her feet from turning down, but I couldn't stand the thought, and I knew Jen would hate it. (I had begun to have secret conversations in my mind with Jennifer that were a great comfort to me.) I turned the issue over and over and finally came up with what I thought might be a solution: we could fix some two-by-fours at the end of her bed and put Jen in big sneakers; if her feet started to curl or drop, they would be restricted by the two-by-fours. I asked if we could try it, and the doctors said yes. So Mike set up the two-by-fours and we got Jen these big, old, ugly gray high-top sneakers—and it worked. The only problem was, as Jennifer finally came out of her coma and began to evolve mentally . . . she fell in love with the sneakers and refused to get rid of them!

The most damaged area of my brain was the part that controls the voice. My doctors were sure I would never speak again. My mother pinned her hopes on the opinion of Dr. Albert Butler, the chair of neurosurgery at Northwestern University's medical school. Immediately after my accident, my uncle Marshall had flown Dr. Butler out from Chicago to look at me and confirm that everything that could be done was being done. Dr. Butler had reviewed my case history and test results with the Concord Hospital doctors, watched as the staff surgeon examined me, and determined that the most updated protocols were being followed. He told my mother I would live and that he felt my prognosis was good. My age was in my favor, and he said he was a strong believer in neuro-rehabilitation. He went on to tell my mother that he had known an anesthesiologist who had suffered a similar injury and had ultimately gone back to work, so anything was possible.

Some years later, Dr. Butler called my mom to catch up. He was astounded to find that I was living on my own all the way across the country, and wanted to know all the details of my recovery.

"It's just like your friend," my mom said.

Confused, he asked, "What friend?"

"You know, the anesthesiologist who successfully returned to work after recovering from a brain injury."

Dr. Butler paused for a moment, and then admitted, "I made that whole thing up."

Maybe I was living on false hope, but it paid off. I waited for Jen to wake up, but I was also persistent. I've always been interested in alternative approaches, so I found myself speaking with psychics, having energy work done on Jen, and I even brought in rose petals to Jen's room that I had been told had healing powers. One of the psychics that I spoke with told me that Jennifer was there, hovering over her body and looking down, trying to decide whether or not she should go back into her body. Evidently, Jen was leaning towards not returning, because her body was so wrecked that she didn't see how she could ever make a go of it.

I about expired on the floor when I heard this. "Well, what can we do?" I asked, on the verge of hysteria. I was told that everyone who had been in the hospital to support her, including myself, should come in and touch and hold her, and provide a safe presence for her. So we did. We did it in shifts. I barely left Jennifer's side; I was allowed to sleep in the day surgery rooms every night but had to get out by five o'clock in the morning so they could use the room. Eventually someone brought me a cot so I could stay in the ICU waiting room. We followed the psychic's instructions for three days, but there was no sign that Jennifer had made a decision, and she still did not wake up.

The doctors suggested bringing in personal items for Jennifer to lure her back into consciousness, so I brought in relics from her old life: our dog, Feather; a bit of her horse's mane; her saddle; even some horse manure; and I played her and Matt's song, "Brown Eyed Girl," over and over; none of that worked either.

I hardly ever bathed while Jennifer was in her coma, but one particular evening, a week after my talk with the psychic, I went back to the rental house to take a bath and wash my hair. I'd been in the same clothes the whole time, except for changing my underwear, but this evening I put on a different sweater that I knew Jen liked. And I thought to myself, "She'd be so pleased to see that I'm wearing something different. This is the perfect day for her to come out of her coma." When I got back to the hospital, a nurse was washing her face. The nurse turned away to the sink—and all of a sudden, Jennifer's left eye opened.

"Her left eye opened!" I exclaimed. Right then, of course, her eye closed before the nurse could see it.

"Oh, Joanne," she said softly, "I know how badly you want this to happen. . . . "

"Listen!" I insisted. "That eye opened!" And right at that moment, her eye opened again.

I went tearing through the halls of the intensive care unit to the waiting room. "Her eye opened!" I yelled, and my mother, Matt, Wendy, and Mike all came thundering down into her room (which was against the rules, of course). When everyone got there, though, both eyes were closed, and they stayed closed for three days. On the third day, she opened that one eye, and it stayed open.

Albert Butler, MD, retired professor of surgery and chief of neurosurgery at Northwestern University

My whirlwind trip from Chicago began with a summons from my dean, a friend of Jennifer's uncle. In "the academic way," he did not ask but told me to go to New Hampshire. He said, "Within the hour, a car will take you to the Fields' private jet." He said they would fly me back to Chicago before morning. They wanted me to judge whether the best that could be done for Jennifer was being done. Was there lethal damage? Bleeding? I checked her cranial pressure. Had it been controlled? How severe was her TBI? These answers would tell me if the thin girl, wreathed in tubes and shadowed by monitors, would survive.

I reviewed her case history, studies, and test results with the Concord Hospital surgeons. I watched as the staff surgeon conducted yet another exam. As the chair of neurosurgery at Northwestern University's school of medicine, I had watched many and I knew the surgeon was following the most up-to-date protocols. I thought, "All that can be done is being done." My conclusion was what the Fields wanted—hoped—to hear, and I told the family this small bit of good news.

As the months went by, I heard from Joanne that "Jenny," as I called her, had started to come around. Later, they came to Chicago, and I was surprised by the amount of Jennifer's recovery. They were shopping for the best rehab facility. Without hesitation, I recommended Henry Betts at the Rehab Institute of Chicago, who was incredible, even fantastic, for providing the extensive rehabilitation that brain and spinal cord injuries demand. I continued to follow Jen's progress via her website, where I viewed her one-woman show. It reinforced my belief in very direct and intensive rehab, which is wonderful, especially for young people.

I have no memory of my months in the coma. However, one psychic told my mother she could see two angels on either side of my bed protecting me and guiding me back. Although many people don't believe in angels or even destiny, I have to believe that, in the midst of this terrible tragedy, certain events speak to angelic presence. Why was Bill the fireman listening to his CB radio at that moment? Why did a small hospital have mannitol on that day? Why was it that the emergency medical technician assigned to the ambulance that day was the only person in the area certified to intubate a patient, a procedure essential for my survival?

I was told we had to start thinking about moving Jennifer to a rehabilitation facility once she stabilized. One of the most painful things I've ever done was visit those rehab centers. When I saw the giant steel and chain apparatus that would be used to lift her into a bathtub, it became crystal clear how severe her accident had been, and how terrible the consequences. I couldn't reconcile the memory of my beautiful daughter sailing over jumps, and this girl who now was crumpled in a wheelchair, facing a seemingly impossible journey. How were we ever going to do this?

Even though I was still in a partial coma, I became stable enough to be moved to a residential rehabilitation unit in Salem, New Hampshire, called Northeast Rehabilitation. It was one of the very few facilities my mom found that would accept me. She applied to dozens of rehabs, out of which only three would admit me because my condition was so severe. They evaluate patients on what is called the Rancho Los Amigos scale. The scale runs from one to ten, indicating the severity of the patient's condition and the likelihood that they will respond to and benefit from treatment. Using that scale, Northeast put me at a three, and since one equates to a vegetable, they did not think I was going to do very well. Luckily, Dr. James Whitlock, the head of Northeast Rehab, gave me a chance. We transferred from Concord Hospital by ambulance and moved in.

Part II

The Journey

Sometimes when you face a wall, you have to turn your focus in a new direction.

"Aftermath"

They come in a flash
Without warning
Visions are the mysteries of life.
I saw a woman crying
As she peered over a girl who lay motionless
I saw a girl laughing
The light came streaming in
The girl started running with
Determination towards nothing familiar
Her vision was a miracle
The girl was a miracle

—Jennifer

Chapter 4

The Early Days

THEY SAY YOU EMERGE FROM A COMA IN STAGES, like a butterfly coming out of a cocoon. Truly, it's not that beautiful, although maybe just as miraculous. My first memory of waking up from my coma is being on the floor of a blue padded room, looking up at my best friend Kristin and an unfamiliar male face. To this day, I think it is the first memory I have of being conscious after the accident.

I was put in the padded room as a safety precaution so that I could flail my legs and arms unconsciously without getting hurt. When I slept, an attendant watched me all night even though my mom was in the room with me. When you come out of a coma, there's a possibility you can become very violent and hurt yourself or someone else. The doctors had told my mother that the more violent a patient is when coming out of a coma, the better the chances for a good recovery. For the last couple of weeks, I had been thrashing around and throwing myself against the sides of the bed, which were also padded. There was hope.

That unfamiliar face I was looking at was Matt's. I had absolutely no idea who he was; someone had to tell me he was my boyfriend. It was a far cry from the classic Hollywood version of coming out of a coma: the patient wakes up with perfect makeup and hair, looks into the eyes of her loved one, and they both get teary. He says to her, "I've been a fool and I'm never going to let you go away again," she smiles, and within a couple of days, they're running through golden fields of wheat.

My reality was that I was lying on a therapy cushion on the floor. Half my head was shaved, the right side of my face was paralyzed, and my right eye was completely shut. I could only smile on my left side. The muscles in my right arm were so badly contracted that no one could move it down, least of all me. At that point in time, I was still being fed through a tube and had a catheter. The things we take for granted—coughing, blowing your nose, sneezing, laughing—I couldn't do. Even today, when I cry, there are no tears.

By the time I entered rehab, I had lost control of virtually every aspect of my life. Later, when I refused to relinquish the awful grey high-top sneakers that saved me

James Whitlock, Jr., MD, neurologist and medical director at Northeast Rehabilitation Hospital, New Hampshire

"Wrecked for life" was the grim prognosis for severe traumatic brain injury (TBI) patients, like Jennifer, more than twenty years ago when she had her accident. Her injuries were deemed too severe to respond to rehab. She wasn't expected to talk or walk again. Ever. Northeast Rehabilitation Hospital was the only rehab hospital to accept her.

What did I see in Jennifer to persuade me to take on her case? To begin with, she had been referred early, soon after her injury. She also showed promising signs: she was responsive to people, showing meaningful signs of interactivity. She was a strong young athlete in great health before her accident and an accomplished horsewoman in equitation and jumping. Also, Jennifer was well educated, highly motivated, and very competitive. Jennifer's gentle but determined nature shone through and grew to be a powerful asset in her recovery.

At the time she came to Northeast Rehab, she was not deeply comatose; she was awakening. TBI patients who are coming out from their long twilight and gaining awareness need quiet—not the confusion and environmental noise of a regular hospital. Home-like rehab settings are safer and more comfortable at that stage. Waking TBI patients can be unfocused and agitated. They can be rambunctious and want to walk but instead they roll out of bed. It's almost humorous—they are not aggressive—it's as if they are intoxicated enough to be falling down.

When Jennifer arrived at Northeast Rehab, she had a feeding tube and she wasn't walking. By the time she left—not more than three months later—she walked unaided, and was talking and remembering her daily life experiences and helping with her own self care. I call her a poster child for what we do. Her progress was accomplished by her immersion in Northeast Rehab's very intense daily routine.

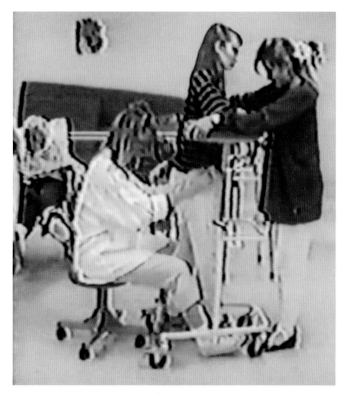

On the high walker, Jennifer's first or second day at Northeast Rehab

from foot drop, I think it was my way of reasserting myself. The old me would have refused to wear those ugly, beat-up shoes, but they became familiar to me when little else was and I found comfort in them.

I couldn't really understand what had happened to me. Questions popped into my head and swam around like small fish in a pool of deep water. I didn't have enough discernment to think, "Something has happened, this is wrong. . . . " My mind was unable to process anything from the past or think about the future; I lived in the moment and nowhere else. My whole world was reduced to that blue padded room and my hospital bed.

My mother lay on a bed near me. I didn't think that was strange at the time; it just seemed right. If you knew my mother, you'd know that nothing could come between her and me. She insisted on staying with me in my room continuously. Both she and my doctor were convinced that her presence would be beneficial to my recovery. The rehab center agreed.

One particular morning, I decided to lie in bed with Jennifer. She seemed restless. She had been thrashing at night and had bruises all over her arms, even though the sides of her bed were padded. She was dozing off and I was looking at her. She hadn't seemed really present and was still lost somewhere inside herself. Suddenly, she opened her eyes and stared back at me. I don't know why I said what I said; I was sure she wouldn't understand or even answer. I asked her, "If you had one wish, what would you wish for?" She looked me right in the eye, and said in a small, halting whisper, "I wish this had never happened." I stared at her in disbelief. Nobody can ever understand how I felt in that moment; I have never been able to talk about it until now. She knew what was going on. We were in this together.

My mother refused to give up hope. In her mind's eye, she still saw me as a beautiful and successful equestrian competitor—and more importantly, she saw me as her whole, normal daughter. I had no horse beneath me, but I was beginning one of the most difficult and important competitions of my life. My mother and I had absolutely no idea of the challenges that lay ahead. We still thought that I would become my old self within a year. Had we truly known how long my recovery would take, we might have become hopelessly discouraged, but our naiveté saved us from giving up.

While Jen was in a coma, I lived in a fantasy world. I still thought of her as that beautiful young woman who could fly around the ring on a horse at world-class shows. As we began the rehab process, though, I was suddenly ripped from that world and thrown into a new reality. The memory of the slings and chains required to get Jen into a bathtub still haunted me. I wasn't even allowed to be in the room when they gave Jen her first bath. I couldn't talk about it at all—I knew if I said anything, I would break down. So I just held everything inside, and kept going.

The rehab process actually began while Jen was still in a coma. There were dangers to watch out for—muscles could atrophy or her blood pressure could spiral out of control. We had watched in horror as, incrementally over the course of the coma, her right arm slowly curled upward until her forearm seemed welded to her bicep. Mike believed he could straighten it, but when he tried it was as if the arm was in a vise and I begged him to stop for fear he would break it. When Jen was transferred to Northeast Rehabilitation, I was told they could pull her arm down a few inches at a time, repeatedly setting it with hard casts, or they could use a device called a Dynasplint. To me the hard casts sounded archaic—I thought Jen-

nifer would hate them—so I chose the Dynasplint, an adjustable metal cast that applied continual gentle pressure. Little by little, her arm straightened.

I had assumed Jen's arm would move normally once it was down and that she might even wave at me. This was not at all the case. Her arm was shockingly limp and inert. Jen being Jen, she would try so hard to move it that her whole body would shake. Regardless of how hard she struggled, she couldn't budge it. Then one day, while she was lying on a therapy table with her arm in an inflatable cast, the therapists asked her to try once again. Her entire body shook, but suddenly this time her index finger moved upward ever so slightly. In that moment I knew if she could do that, she could do anything.

We even tried therapeutic riding, with aides in front, in back, and on either side of Jen as she sat atop a gentle horse. You could see glimmers of the rider she had

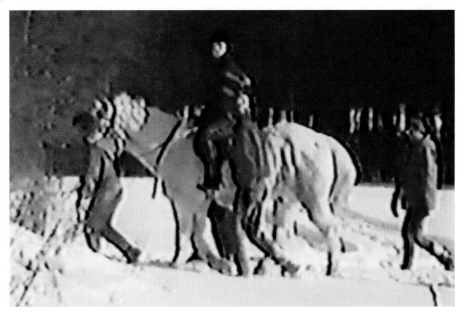

Riding a therapy horse at Northeast Rehab

been—she reflexively tried to move her hands to take the reins—but she had lost any real sense of what she was supposed to do. It was heart-breaking to watch.

At the forefront of my mind, I maintained a vision of myself as healed—walking, talking, and having fun with my friends. I know it's hard to believe, but at the be-

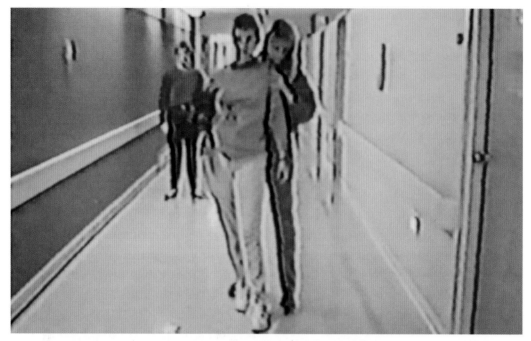

Learning to walk again at Northeast Rehab

ginning of my recovery, I almost never got depressed. The therapies took up most of my days and my mother always made sure I was busy or distracted by a card game, another therapy, or spending time with friends and relatives. Because of the damage to my brain, I wasn't aware that I had changed; in that early period of recovery, I couldn't remember how I was before the accident. My history as a determined competitor was still lost inside me, waiting to be called upon.

I have no memory of the few months that preceded my accident. I can't remember riding my horses during that time. My mother told me that I'd placed third at Madison Square Garden the previous November and had taken the champion title at the Washington Horse Show in Maryland in the Junior Jumper division. I had been so successful but couldn't remember any of it. I was frustrated beyond belief at the loss of those memories, but there was nothing I could do. Even today they are still lost to me except for pictures and videos of the event. I want to remember them so badly that I sometimes feel like I actually do.

Looking back, I don't recall much about that early time period at Northeast Rehab either. It's like watching a fictional movie that I didn't live. I see myself on the screen, staggering down the hallway with a therapist holding me up with a therapy belt, and even today I don't remember being that girl. As I progressed and went from my bed, to a wheelchair, to walking with a cane, I really wasn't present in my own body. I was like a robot following commands, but my brain was not yet connected. There are also some videos from back then and when I think back on that period of time, I don't know if I have actual memories, or if I'm just remembering the videos.

Today, there are bits and pieces that I do recall. I remember, so clearly, turning over in my bed at Northeast Rehab, and thinking, "Where am I? What's going on? What happened?" And I remember, later, how arduous it was transferring to my wheelchair, even with help, and going to the bathroom, and how impossible it was to wash my face. I had followed the rigorous Erno Lazlo regime that required splashing my face thirty times with hot water. I wasn't able to do that. But finally, one day my mother said, "Let's get back to the face routine." She held me at the sink and helped me—I used my left hand and she stood behind me and used her right, and we splashed my face thirty times!

I was so excited when Dr. Whitlock came to me and said it was time to remove the feeding tube. We had two options. One was to go to the hospital and have it removed in a surgical procedure. The second was for the doctor to just pull the tube out in her room. I couldn't bear the thought of Jennifer going back to the hospital and being put under, so I opted for Dr. Whitlock pulling it out. When he wound the tubing several times around his hand and braced his foot against the bed, I had second thoughts.

As the cord tightened, a look of horror and pain crossed Jennifer's face. Suddenly the cord popped out and I saw the ball on the other side of the tubing that had caused the resistance. "Yikes," I said to myself, thinking Jennifer would never remember, but to this day she still brings it up! "There," said Dr. Whitlock brightly, "that's out! Now she can start on pureed food."

I'd been on a feeding tube for so long that pureed meals truly seemed like dinner at a five-star restaurant. I'd blissfully eat bowls and bowls of pureed peas, chicken, pears, and carrots, until one day, my mother saw me eating my fifth helping and said, "Jennifer . . . maybe you shouldn't eat so much."

I kept shoveling food into my mouth as I whispered, "I . . . was . . . in . . . a . . . co . . . maaaa . . . not . . . eating . . . I . . . must . . . have . . . lost . . . weight."

My mom said, "Well. Not quite."

I guess the tube feeding provided more calories than I'd thought. Evidently I'd actually gained a little weight while in the coma.

In March of 1993, five months after the accident, Jennifer was able to become an outpatient, and we moved into a rented house next to the rehab facility. I had to work as hard at relearning who my daughter was as she had to work relearning certain tasks. One evening, I was helping Jennifer get ready for bed. I buttoned only two or three of the buttons on her pajamas, and I'd moved on to the next bit of preparation when Jennifer whispered in that same halting voice, "Why aren't you doing up all of my buttons?"

I panicked. I had never known my child liked all of her buttons done up! After all these years, how could I not know something like that about my child?! Wracking my brain, I tried to remember Jennifer with all of her buttons done up. I couldn't for the life of me picture it, but I carefully buttoned each one. And she said, "Thank you!"

Three or four months later, we were getting ready for bed again, and I did up all of her buttons. To my surprise, she stopped me and said, "Why are you doing up all of my buttons?" I later found out that certain ritualistic and compulsive behaviors can be very common with people with brain injuries, and that's what I'd been seeing in those months of buttoning.

Each bit of work that Jennifer did amazed me, and we often had to start from the simplest places. On day one, Jen couldn't hold her head up, because she'd been in bed so long that her neck muscles had atrophied. The physical therapists put her in a special head-injury wheelchair that had a high back and a head brace. I didn't think she needed it. I kept saying, "Of course she can hold her head up!" The therapists removed the brace, and her head just flopped over. I couldn't get it into my mind that a head injury could have all of these repercussions. I couldn't believe that it was really my daughter who couldn't hold her own head up. We tried a Thomas-type cervical collar for a bit and a week of physical therapy until finally Jen was able to hold her head up on her own.

I kept asking the physical therapists how long they thought Jen's recovery would take, expecting them to say "a few months." Everyone was very kind to me when they explained that it might take longer because Jen's injury was so severe. Something stopped me from pressing for a more definitive answer; I secretly told myself it might take a year.

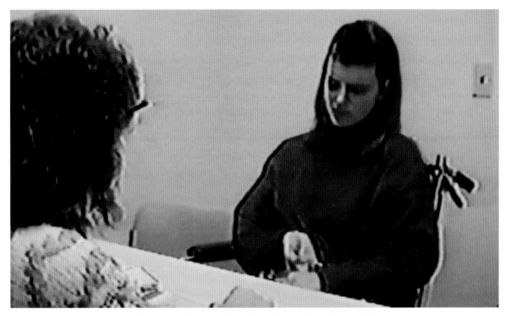

Working with a speech therapist at Northeast Rehab

I learned, bit by bit, that Jennifer simply wouldn't be able to do all of the standard things she'd done before. During one occupational therapy session, the therapist asked her to fit a triangle-shaped peg into the corresponding hole. She couldn't do it, but I just couldn't accept that. I sent friends and family shopping for early learning toys and games. I sat her down and said to her—like an adult—"Jennifer, please don't be offended by the toys meant for two- and three-year-olds. A lot of the things we're going to do together are going to be like when you were a baby. But we have to start here." She and I would drill and drill with them until she finally got it. Jen and I are both competitive by nature, so when we returned for the next appointment and Jen was able to complete all of the tasks, we delighted in the therapist's amazement.

My mother helped me see my progress in terms of "yesterday versus today." She was always there to remind me of what I had accomplished today that I was not able to accomplish yesterday. She helped me to define what came next, and she always made sure my spirits were up.

I needed the routine and structure that my mother helped provide. I felt comforted and safe with the consistency. I have learned that, with a head injury or a neurological disorder of any kind, it's very important to give the patient a feeling of safety; I was no exception to that rule.

I also desperately needed and wanted people to treat me as if I would fully recover. Like my mother, I didn't want the thought that I might not be the person I had been to enter my mind. It might have been a form of denial, but I was determined to return to life as it had been before the accident. Only later did I discover that I would never be exactly the same as I once was.

Late in February of 1993, we were told that we'd be able to take Jennifer on an outing to the mall. This was a huge moment for all of us—it was her first excursion! I had decided to get my hair done, so I went to the salon while Kristin and Matt took Jennifer around the mall in her wheelchair. I was getting my color touched up when Kristin and Matt burst into the salon with Jennifer. It was the first time I'd seen my daughter outside of the confines of the rehab facility and in a public environment—and what I saw was really heartbreaking for me.

There she was in a wheelchair with half of her head shaved, one eye closed, and very little expression on her face. I had to try extremely hard to not burst into tears while Matt and Kristin happily told me about the wonderful time they'd had, taking her from store to store. "For goodness' sake, Joanne," I thought, "concentrate on what is great about this situation. This is a huge step forward." I smiled wanly, and told Matt and Kristin that I would meet them in the mall restaurant when my hair was finished.

Holding back tears, I watched them leave. The hairdresser, a young woman, looked at me in the mirror as they left and said, "How sad!" That was a knife in my heart. It made it all the more real.

I had to relearn *everything*—how to walk, how to talk, even, in some cases, how to be polite in social situations again. I went through the entire process of voice development, like a young child. I would blurt things out like a little kid in the truth of the moment—with pure, innocent, child-like honesty. No one was ever sure what would come out of my mouth. I'd see something or think of something, and out the words would come, without the slightest thought that I might be embarrassing or hurting someone. I remember once being in my hospital room with a lot of my family members and Matt. I looked at Matt closely, and blurted out, "Matt, did we ever have sex?" He was mortified, but I thought it was a reasonable question, since I honestly couldn't remember.

Chapter 5

THE ROAD TO RECOVERY

In March of 1993, I received a phone call from my friend Wendy. "Joanne," she said, "I don't know if you would be interested, but there's a woman named Martha Estin in Marblehead, Massachusetts. She's an alternative practitioner working with brain injury victims, and she's become hugely successful."

"Are you kidding?!" I exclaimed. "Yes! I would be more than interested." I took down Martha's number. Later that week, as we pulled up in front of Martha's company, Brainworks, I thought to myself, "Please, please let this be something wonderful for Jennifer. Please let this be something that reconnects her brain." We got Jen into her wheelchair and went in.

Martha greeted us at the door. She was a small, blond-haired woman with more energy than five people put together. As we felt out our new surroundings, Martha told us about her son, Sarge. He had experienced hundreds of seizures since his

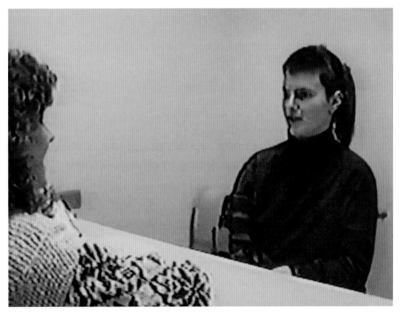

Out of the wheelchair and beginning to improve

birth, and Martha had developed several different therapies and techniques to help him. She had been successful, and Sarge was now seizure-free and teaching under his own company, Active Healing.

Martha explained that from birth we develop physically and neurologically by using our senses of sight, hearing, and touch to understand our environment and function within it. Her program of exercises helped me to re-experience the basic developmental stages that infants go through and to retrain my brain in the same way that I would have self-trained as a child learning to crawl for the first time.

The first therapy Martha taught us involved "cross patterning." Jennifer lay on a table on her back, and three different people moved her arms, legs, and head simultaneously to simulate normal walking: we moved her right arm and left leg while turning her head towards her raised arm, then moved her left arm and right leg and turned her head the other way. Martha explained that cross patterning would help repair pathways between the left and right sides of Jennifer's brain so that signals controlling the nervous system could pass freely. I couldn't believe it! Martha was actually saying that her therapy would reconnect Jennifer's brain and body!

Cross patterning helped me tremendously because it reoriented me with my surroundings. In the following months with Martha, I crawled for so long that I covered every square inch of my house and ended up with permanent rug burn!

Martha's next therapy was to string Jennifer upside down. I watched in shock as Martha deftly wrapped plastic mesh bands around Jen's ankles and used the bands to hang her from a wooden ladder that was suspended horizontally. To my horror, Martha spun Jennifer in a wildly circular motion—first one way, then the other—for what seemed like a very, very long time. She explained that this particular technique was to help Jennifer's equilibrium. I just nodded. Martha knew what she was doing. I hoped!

The next step was to have Jennifer, still hanging from the ladder, read various flashcards that Martha placed on the ground underneath her. This was to help connect her eyes with her brain. Amazingly, Jennifer did not seem to mind the spinning exercise. Maybe she could feel that it was making a difference.

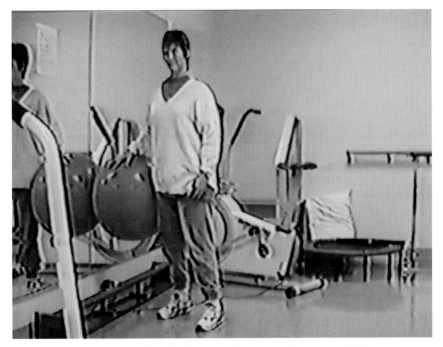

Working with a physioball at Rehabilitation Institute of Chicago

The final therapy for her on that first day was "rebreathing." The process, also known as hypercapnia, involves rebreathing one's own exhaled carbon dioxide and can actually increase oxygenation to the brain by as much as sixty percent. Increasing the blood level of carbon dioxide triggers deep breathing and vasodilation (dilation of blood vessels that bring oxygen to the brain), and the combination of the two dramatically increases the oxygen in the cerebral blood flow. All Jen had to do was breath into a modified oxygen mask. I could actually see Jennifer's eyes brighten and color come into her cheeks as she breathed into the mask.

In May of 1993, it was time to take the next step. We made the switch from Northeast Rehabilitation to the Rehabilitation Institute of Chicago, where my brother lived. I felt we'd reached a point where Jennifer needed to move on, and the Rehabilitation Institute was said to be the best in the United States. Jen had also developed a tremor in her left arm. Her right arm was almost useless and now her left arm was compromised, and I felt it was time for her to try some different tactics. We could continue with most of Martha's therapies in Chicago.

We left Northeast Rehab and moved to Chicago for treatment at the Rehabilitation Institute of Chicago (known as RIC) in the spring of 1993. I was excited. I thought moving to Chicago was going to be great for me, not only because it was a new chapter in my recovery, but because my Uncle Marshall and his family were there. My mom and I stayed at his apartment in the city on Michigan Avenue, and every Friday he'd pick us up and drive us out to their house in Lake Forest so we could spend the weekend with them. During the week we spent every day at RIC learning new exercises and therapies that would help me reconnect with my body.

My family was wonderful. They treated me like there was nothing wrong with me—taking me out to dinner, doing crossword puzzles with me, and playing cards. The reality of my doing a crossword puzzle was that Uncle Marsh would read the question to me, I would pretend to think, and he would come up with the answer, and say, "Great, Jen!" That semblance of normalcy helped me immensely.

Even with family life helping me along, there were good days and bad days. The good days were filled with small victories. One task I remember clearly was opening clothespins with my right hand, and then clasping them onto an upright ruler. My right arm was still mostly paralyzed from the coma, when it had been curled up tight against my chest; trying to open one simple clothespin was, for me, like climbing Mount Everest. My fingers didn't work correctly and I had very little strength in my hand; my muscles were working against the movement I wanted to make. When I could finally, slowly, open the clothespin, stretch my arm shakily above my head to clamp each pin on the ruler, I felt like I'd won a competition. Each succeeding clothespin clamped higher was an additional blue ribbon.

Looking back, I realize that the physical therapists were targeting specific muscles and strengthening them individually, but at the time, it was often tedious, boring, and extremely tiring. I also remember having to press a large physioball against the wall with my hip and simultaneously lift the opposite leg and take a step forward and then backward, sometimes up onto a platform. I thought this would be easy, but when I couldn't even lift my toe off the floor, I realized that I still had so much work to do, and the rebuilding of my body would take far longer than I had ever imagined. Still, I always retained the inner resolve to master every task that was given to me. I felt it just had to be exactly right.

Even as we began a new chapter in Jen's recovery in Chicago, I was determined to try anything and everything that I thought might help. In May, we went to a local

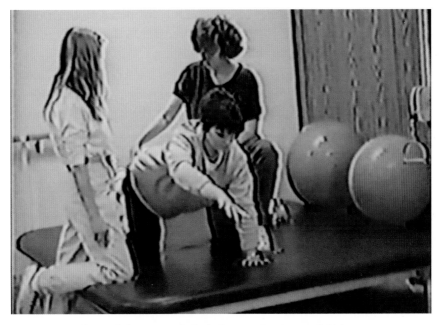

Physical therapy at Rehabilitation Institute of Chicago

healer from Sri Lanka. He'd married the mayor's daughter, and was living and practicing in Chicago. Somehow I thought that since he had married the mayor's daughter, he must be reliable and good at what he did.

He began by explaining that he would put his hands on different parts of Jennifer's body to find the negative energy. That made sense. Then he told us that once he found those pockets of negative energy, he would burp to release the bad energy. I felt my eyes getting wide with disbelief, but there we were.

He put Jen's feet in warm water and began to lay hands on her. Soon came the burp. Then another burp. Uh-oh, I thought. Another burp, louder and longer. And then the worst thing happened—laughter bubbled up inside me, and I couldn't control myself. I fled the room and buried my face in a curtain in the waiting area, hoping he wouldn't hear me laughing. After a short time I walked back in, pretending nothing had happened. He declared that they'd had a great session. I don't know how much it helped, but we did return a few times.

After we had the first session with the healer, I thought about why so many trainers had told me they loved working with Jen back in her competitive riding days: she did exactly what they instructed and never questioned them. She was an ideal student and had extraordinary focus. It occurred to me that it was probably *her ability to focus that helped her to not become distracted by the ever-increasing volume of the burps, whereas I completely lost it. Jennifer was so intent on getting well, she didn't notice his bizarre behavior.*

Our time in Chicago was very productive, between the services at RIC, alternative therapies, and time spent with family. We were finally able to return home in May although we traveled back and forth to Chicago for the next year to consult with doctors and therapists.

Laura Tolman, Jennifer's best friend in high school

Jennifer and I were best friends in high school. We were always together. I was a boarding student and Jennifer was a day student. She would get out of her car in the morning, walk to my dorm, wait for me to get dressed, and then we'd go to breakfast. We didn't have many classes together, but every free moment we had at school, we spent together. Looking back, neither of us can quite remember how we met—we just became inseparable.

On the day of Jen's accident, her boyfriend Matt was coming up from Connecticut and the plan was that I would go home with her after school and cook dinner for them. But it turned out that I had to stay at school and give a tour to prospective students, so she hopped into her car alone and drove off into the snowstorm.

The next thing I knew, I was being rushed to the headmaster's office. I had no idea what was going on—I thought I was in trouble. The headmaster sat me down and told me gently that Jen had been in a very bad accident, and that they weren't sure how she was doing.

I froze in place. All that came out of my teenage mouth was, "But she's my best friend." I kept saying it, over and over. I couldn't conceive of my best friend in high school being in a life-threatening situation. Another day student had seen the accident while driving in, and he'd run through the halls trying to find me. That's when the school administrators pulled me into the office and shut the door. No one knew what had really happened, but a rumor quickly started up about Jennifer not surviving the accident. I just sat there in the office, frozen.

Later my friend, Walker, and I sat outside the school in the dark, waiting for Matt to arrive. We were left with the task of telling him what had happened. He didn't believe us at first. I still couldn't quite believe it either.

The next day, Jen's advisor told me Jen was in a coma and asked me to visit and talk to her. He volunteered to drive me back and forth.

The environment at school was odd after Jen's accident. I was in a haze without my best friend. Kids made insensitive remarks. I don't think anybody fully grasped the magnitude of the event; we were just too young. Even months later when I visited Jen at the rehab center and watched her being assisted with everything, I couldn't really comprehend what had happened.

Jen did come back and walk with us at graduation. We were supposed to process in alphabetical order but they put her at the front and we walked together. Everyone had red roses, but Jen and I carried yellow ones—it was very special.

Jen and I fell out of touch after that. The rest of us graduated and went our own ways—to college, to programs abroad. A few years later, Jen's friend Mike approached me in a café and told me how abandoned Jen had felt. We'd all just disappeared after high school, without giving much thought to anyone left behind, and it was really hard for Jen.

Eventually, I went to nursing school. As we were choosing our final rotations, I realized that I wanted to try working in rehab. It was only once I started working with accident victims and other patients that I understood how severe Jen's accident had really been. I don't think I would have made that choice of career without having known Jen. She changed the course of my life.

I moved back to the area after getting married, and one day Jen and I ran into each other. We took the opportunity to grab lunch, and managed to pick up right where we left off. Jen was a wonderful person to begin with, but after we rekindled our friendship, I saw how much the accident had matured her. It's incredible how much she's progressed. Every time we get together, she's doing a bit better; I'm so glad we've gotten back in touch.

My original plan before the accident had been to graduate early from the Dublin School so I could compete in Europe at several equestrian competitions there. Because of this plan, I had completed most of my high school credits before the night of the accident. The school was incredibly understanding and allowed me to graduate with the rest of my class in June of 1993. When the day came, I was incredibly excited. I was surrounded by family and friends—I had made it! My dad and my stepmother came from New York, my grandmother came from Washington, D.C., and Matt came from Connecticut. I was happy he made the effort to come. I hoped this meant Matt was going to be back in my life again.

Watching Jen graduate was surreal, and in many ways, bittersweet. We'd been to hell and back, and yet there she was, walking down the aisle in her beautiful white dress. Her friend Laura helped her on stage to receive her diploma. I could hear a buzz in the audience as everyone grasped what this moment truly meant.

Jennifer stood on stage glowing as each member of the class was called up. At the moment her name was finally called and she was able to step forward on her own to receive her diploma, the whole auditorium erupted with cheers and applause. Jen basked in the glory as I dissolved into sobs. I couldn't stop crying for the duration of the ceremony, and I left still wracked with tears. In hindsight, I think that day may have been the first time that I really let myself fully feel the depth of my pain—and the first time, too, that I could experience the beginning of Jen's transcendence.

I was so happy to be surrounded by my friends and to feel their love and support. I couldn't get over the fact that I was standing on stage with my classmates, going through Commencement only six and a half months after my accident. And yet there I was. The effort I had to put into each step was immense, but worth it all. I focused with all my might on the ground and prayed that I wouldn't fall. I didn't. And it didn't escape me how perfect and necessary it was to have a break from the intensity of my rehabilitation— to have, just for a moment, the normal life I craved.

Chapter 6

Falling Off the Horse

AS A COMPETITIVE HORSEBACK RIDER I trained diligently every day. It was never easy, and I fell many, many times along the way. One of my worst falls was in the practice warm-up at the Del Mar International Horse Show in California in the spring of 1992.

It was my first international show, and I was really feeling the pressure. As I approached the first jump, the sun was setting. I saw the jump, but Swanny must have seen only shadow because she took off too early. Her hooves caught the back rail, and I was catapulted out of the saddle. I landed hard. Dazed, I had to be helped out of the ring.

Miraculously, Swanny wasn't hurt at all. I didn't break any bones, but I was sore enough that as I went back to the hotel with packages of ice, I was sure the competition was over for me. The next day though, I felt better so I went back to the ring. Swanny and I entered the speed class, a jumping course based on how fast you can complete the course without knocking any rails down. We came in second.

As I look back on it, I find it somewhat amazing that I had no fear of getting back on the horse. Perseverance, drive, and my love of competition always put me back in the saddle. My trainer had told me that the Olympics were in my future, and that goal was always in my mind, helping me to push through. Every fall or mistake I made was a step towards that ultimate goal.

Once I got back home from Chicago, it was inevitable that I would ask my mother to take me down to the barn. Approaching from the path, I could see my horse Swanny sticking her head out of a small window in the front of the barn. As we got closer, I could see she recognized me, and at that moment pieces of the puzzle started flooding back. I remembered being in the ring, clearing jumps, and racing against the clock.

I was completely overcome with emotion as I reached up and touched Swanny's nose. I had this overwhelming feeling of excitement at the thought of riding again. Swanny and I stared at each other, and I knew that we both longed to compete together. I could almost hear her hooves thundering toward the last jump and the

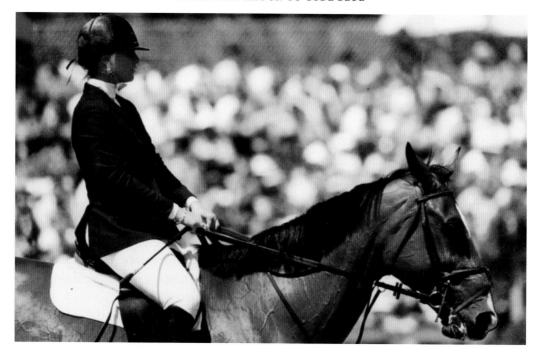

Riding Swan Lake in 1992, a few months before the accident

crowd erupting as we sped through the timers. I turned to look at my mom, and the look in her eyes said it all: that was never going to happen.

My doctors thought getting back on a horse was a bad idea; looking back, I can see that it was a little bit crazy, and at the least, risky. Riding had been my life, though—it was all I knew. My mother understood, because it had been her life too. She was worried, but she believed it held a key to speeding up my recovery, and so she agreed to let me try.

In the end, it didn't matter how supportive and encouraging people were, or whether my mom said she could see the old rider that I had been. Once I was back on a horse, I couldn't feel it. I had no sensory memory, no knowledge of how to control the huge animal using my arms and legs. My reaction time was slow and my legs were too weak to grip Swanny's sides.

I fell.

I was sitting in the kitchen talking on the phone when someone came running from the barn, yelling, "Jen fell!" An overwhelming feeling of panic descended on me as I went running down to the barn. I saw Jen's trainer kneeling beside her with Jen's head on her lap.

"I think she's okay," she said, "but her eyes rolled back in her head after she fell."

"Someone call for an ambulance!" I screamed as I ran towards Jennifer.

I could see when I reached her that her eyes were tracking, and she seemed to be all right. "Jennifer, how do you feel?" I asked, hoping that the ambulance wouldn't be necessary.

"Okay," she said weakly. I stared at her long and hard and decided that we really did need to go to the hospital. The ambulance arrived, and I got in beside her. The whole event pitched me toward an emotional place I hadn't been to in a long while, and sitting in the ambulance, I realized that I was shaking.

The doctors at the hospital checked her out and said that no damage had been done. They did, however, reiterate that riding would be extremely risky for her. As I stared at them, I thought, they just don't understand. Jennifer has got to be able to ride again if she is going to make a recovery. At that point I still believed that riding was her ticket to getting back to normal. In my mind, if she could ride, that meant she was well.

When I got home from my latest trip to the hospital, I went to my room and thought about what had happened. I believed that I needed to be able to be on a horse again to feel normal, so several days later, I decided to make another go of it. The risk was completely lost on me, even as doctors told me not to do it, because I believed the reward would be so great.

Determined, I got back up on Swanny, but when I fell a second time the stubborn confidence I'd had gave way to fear. I was terrified that if I continued my riding, I would eventually fall on my head, reinjure my brain, and be worse off than I already was. Riding had been my biggest dream—my *only* dream—and now, it was gone.

I felt numb and completely lost. I thought of turning to Matt, but he was becoming frustrated and resentful over how long it was taking me to recover and was starting to leave more and more time between visits. Eventually, he stopped coming at all.

The funny thing is, we never actually broke up. There was no big confrontational argument. The words "it's over" were never spoken, and so it didn't matter how many months passed without seeing him; I had it in my head that he was still my boyfriend. I was completely convinced that he would come through the door, and that we would go right back to laughing and joking while driving around in his Le

Baron. That fantasy didn't change until his number stopped working. I called his father only to learn that Matt was married and had a daughter. That was devastating for me—I had been waiting for him to come back, and he never would. First I lost my riding, my center, and then Matt, my boyfriend. I had to dig deep to keep going.

I could see that Jennifer was heartbroken and sinking into a depression. I decided I had to find an activity to distract her that would hopefully somehow make up for this devastating loss. I knew that she needed something else besides the endless hours of hard work that she put into her therapies every day. It occurred to me that driving again would be great for Jen—she would be able to regain some independence—so I called the driving instructor at Crotched Mountain Rehabilitation Center in Greenfield, New Hampshire, and set up an appointment. He took her out driving several times, and then announced that he thought she would be okay on the road.

The day after the instructor cleared Jen to drive, we'd planned to go to the Brattleboro Retreat in Vermont for a therapy appointment. "Great," I thought, "I can let Jennifer drive!"

To say the drive was hair-raising would be an understatement. I had to keep grabbing the wheel so we wouldn't go off the road. Jennifer thought she was driving perfectly and was so happy, but I feared for my life and hers. Her depth perception was way off. I knew she wasn't ready to drive, and I felt terrible. I realized I had to take yet another thing away from my daughter. When we got home, I worked up the courage to disappoint my child and she burst into tears.

"Is there anything I'm going to be able to do?" she cried. It hurt to look at her and know that I didn't have an answer.

Riding and competing were gone from my life, and I thought my social life was gone as well. My energy was severely limited. I believed that my whole life was slowly drifting away. Nothing felt permanent anymore.

With my old life of riding, competing, and relationships behind me, I made my recovery my main purpose. My mother, who was my biggest advocate, always distracted me with new therapies she had researched, and let absolutely nothing get between me and getting well.

As I began to regain some of the basic skills I lost in the accident, I was able to focus all of my energy on recovery. As I got better, my strength and energy grew.

I didn't think about the future—and I definitely didn't think about the past. Life was just about accomplishing the next task at hand, whether it was staying on the balance beam, cross patterning, or walking on the driveway. My desire to get better became the driving force that got me through each day. Whenever I saw any improvement, I would be eager to begin again the next day. This was my life for the moment, I told myself, but one day things would be different.

As Jennifer's recovery progressed, she and I began to have typical mother-daughter tiffs. They were never anything big, but she was a young woman and I was her mother and, of course, we didn't always see eye to eye—"Jennifer, you're not doing this exercise right. . . ." "But, Mom!" Once we left Chicago and started to do rehab in our home back in New Hampshire, Mike Martin became an indispensable third party.

Mike had been a horse trainer before he became the caretaker of my property. He was able to see Jennifer's body in a way that I couldn't. So he stepped in to implement all the therapies on a daily basis.

It was thrilling, watching her progress with Mike. I converted the great room in our house into a rehab room, and we'd get exercises from the Rehabilitation Institute of Chicago for them to work on. Within a week, she'd master them, and I'd call back looking for more exercises. The therapists in Chicago would say, "There's no way Jennifer could've mastered that in a week!" but she always did. I was also able to recreate Martha Estin's therapy room in our space, and we followed Martha's program every day. For the next year and a half, Martha came once or twice a month until Jen was so much better that she was able to apply cross patterning to her walking.

In Chicago the red physioball had been one of my greatest challenges. When I went home I practiced every day with Mike. I visualized myself lifting my leg and placing it easily on a step, the same way I used to envision myself clearing a jump with Swanny. I was determined to master this small skill and one day, I did. The thrill wasn't complete until I knew my mother had called the therapists in Chicago and told them what I'd done. They had a hard time believing it. Mike and I were thrilled. Every accomplishment was a step forward.

Mike Martin, Fields' property caretaker and friend

Six months after the accident Jennifer left rehab and returned home to continue her therapies. Mrs. Field believed one would enhance another, so Jennifer had multiple therapies and kept adding them.

Not a day went by that we didn't engage in something—Martha's program of rebreathing, cross-creeping and crawling, hanging and spinning from a ladder, Dr. Padula's eye exercises, specific exercises from the rehab, or therapists coming to the house who specialized in different treatments. There was always work to be done. One person couldn't do it all; we had to trade off and take turns. I coached Jen and encouraged her when necessary, and I drove thousands of miles with her and Mrs. Field to specific therapists. When we weren't driving, we were working. None of us had another life. Mrs. Field never took a day off.

What kept us going were Jen's improvements: first little itty-bitty things, and then those little things got even better. And we made it fun. We had to keep laughing and finding things to focus on and laugh at while Jen worked and worked. She used to watch a movie, *The Cutting Edge*, over and over while she cross-crawled around the great room. She watched it so many times we could all recite dialogue from it!

We would start at ten o'clock in the morning and work until one. Then we'd eat lunch and go right back to work from two o'clock until four. It was tedious and repetitive: the same things over and over and over—creeping, crawling, physioball, spinning from the ladder, eye exercises. We joked and teased to keep ourselves entertained and to help Jen get her sense of humor back.

We were happy and laughing; we had the constant stimulation of friends and family helping. Having a team behind you is important and necessary. And we all saw Jen's improvement—our hard work was paying off.

Silly, silly stuff made us laugh. Once, we went out to dinner after Jen had gotten a massage and her muscles were all loose. When she came out of the restroom, she was walking kind of at an angle, headed straight for a plate glass window! Mrs. Field and I just froze. When Jen made it to our table without falling, we all collapsed laughing. Another time during a drive, Jennifer gasped really loudly, and Mrs. Field and I froze again, waiting for the worst.

"What?"

"I forgot my gum!"

Chapter 7

GETTING BACK ON THE HORSE

MY MOTHER TRIED HER BEST TO MAINTAIN some semblance of normalcy for me. We always used to take a trip to Los Angeles every year to visit family, friends, and my mother's former nanny. In July of 1993, we decided I was ready to make the trip again. We invited my friend Kristin and flew out to the West Coast.

It was a giant step forward to be able to restart our tradition of an annual trip to Los Angeles. The girls had a great time, but it was obviously hard for Jennifer to navigate in the real world. Everyone kept talking about how great she seemed to be doing, but the reality was that she was struggling. Jen had trouble walking, communicating, getting in and out of cars—she had trouble doing almost everything.

Curiously, Jennifer was oblivious to the impact she had on people and unaware of her surroundings. Her balance was off and each step was halting, but she was unaware of it. One night at our favorite restaurant, I watched her totter back from the bathroom, swaying from side to side between tables, almost losing her balance at every step. My impulse was to run over and help her, but I didn't. I could see how people were staring at her. It was a real eye opener for me and incredibly hard to watch. I struggled to hang on to my belief that she would be healed. In that moment I felt very alone and fearful, but I clung to the promise that I had made to myself: I would find the therapies to make her better.

That was our first trip away, and as our vacation progressed I became anxious to get back to the familiar surroundings of our home in New Hampshire. We needed to continue our work with Martha Estin and look for new therapies.

Once I got home, my brain played a cruel trick on me. "You're home now, and everything will be back to normal!" it whispered. But Jennifer was not anywhere close to normal, and that was very hard for me to accept. That night, as I lay in my bed feeling extremely depressed, a diaphanous human shape appeared at the end of my bed. As I watched, not questioning, not fearful, a voice said, "Go downstairs, get your books, and start reading."

I knew exactly which books to get. I didn't question what the shape was or why it was there. Somehow, I just knew I was being instructed to get my alternative health books. I had been interested in alternative medical practices for several years and had acquired quite a library. Without a second thought, I went downstairs and grabbed as many of those books as I could carry. I knew I had been pointed in a new direction toward Jennifer's ultimate recovery.

I stacked the books on the rug beside my bed and opened one by Dr. Carlton Fredericks, whose work I quite respected. In it there was a story about a young boy who had had a stroke. Dr. Fredericks, along with a Swiss doctor, had formulated a medicinal tonic to help the boy regain his brain function. The boy took the tonic for several months with extraordinary results. "Wow, there it is," I thought. "I have to get this tonic, and Jennifer will be on her way!"

When I woke up the next morning, I couldn't wait to go downstairs and find a phone number to call Dr. Fredericks. I finally found a home number. Dr. Fredericks' wife picked up, and I held my breath.

She told me that Dr. Fredericks had passed away some time earlier. I was devastated.

Despite my disappointment, I managed to ask his widow if she knew of anyone producing the tonic that he had formulated. She told me about a woman named Dr. Patricia Kane, but she wasn't sure what she did or where she lived. She thought she might be practicing in New Jersey. I knew I had to track her down.

I became an expert at tracking people. It wasn't easy back then; I didn't have a computer at the time and the Internet was still in its early stages. I used 4-1-1 and operators like people today use Google. I found Dr. Kane, who was indeed living in New Jersey, and managed to persuade her to come stay with us in New Hampshire and treat Jennifer.

Dr. Kane, whose specialty was nutrition, was very different from other specialists with whom we'd worked. Sadly, she did not have Dr. Fredericks' formula, but she helped in other ways. During the time she was with us, she changed Jen's diet and showed us how some foods could be counterproductive to recovery, like—to our horror—garlic. Jen loved garlic, and I was used to adding it to a lot of the foods we ate. Dr. Kane roasted a whole batch of garlic for Jen to eat one night, and I watched my daughter's speech and movements slow like a windup toy running down. That was the beginning of a new way of thinking about food and its effects on the brain.

At Dr. Kane's recommendation, we decided to look into craniosacral therapy at the Upledger Institute in Palm Beach Gardens, Florida. Craniosacral therapy involves regulating the flow of cerebrospinal fluid through therapeutic touch, and Dr. Upledger was one of the leading authorities in the practice. An osteopath, he had observed that spinal fluid moved and flowed rhythmically, and he was able to control body energy with his hands by manipulating that spinal fluid. We heard he'd had great success in helping many people with head injuries.

We took the plunge. In March of 1994, we went to the Upledger Institute for a two-week brain injury workshop, where Jennifer worked with several therapists each day. We were in a group of about fifteen other people with head injuries, ranging from infants to adults. At least two of the participants regaled us with stories of their improvements—how when they started with Dr. Upledger they couldn't walk or talk, and now they could.

Hearing about the successes of others, Jen asked me, "Why don't I have these giant leaps forward?"

"You have made great progress," I told her, "and you will continue to make progress. We will find the therapies that will enable you to advance—inch by inch by inch."

That concept stayed with me. In the beginning, I had been so naive that I had thought we'd find a miracle cure and immediately solve everything. Now, though, I knew with all my heart that we would get there inch by inch by inch. More important than my believing it, Jennifer believed it. Her determination and drive was the force for her recovery. She simply refused to give up.

Chapter 8

Inch by Inch by Inch

After we finished the two-week Upledger program, we returned home to continue the core therapies Jennifer used every day. She worked very hard with Mike, and we all started to see real improvement. I felt that the addition of the alternative therapies really made a difference.

On one of our trips back to Chicago we met with Jen's physiatrist, a doctor specializing in physical medicine and rehabilitation. The doctor asked Jennifer to walk up and down a long hallway while she watched her. Seeing Jennifer walk through the doctor's eyes, I realized she looked a little like Quasimodo. Nonetheless, she was walking and I said to the doctor, "Look how much she has improved! We are doing so many alternative treatments to help her."

The doctor turned to me, looked me right in the eye, and said, "Joanne, don't you realize how severe your daughter's brain injury is? She will never get any better than this." I dug my fingernails into the palms of my hands to keep from crying. I could not accept what she said on any level. It was devastating. That night my godchild Wendy said to me, "Don't listen to that doctor! Jennifer is going to get well. You can do it!" In that moment I resolved it would happen—and we were off and running again.

I knew I couldn't quit. No matter how tired I was or how discouraged I got, I had to keep going. There was no thought of ever giving up. Ever. I had to become a person again. There was never a moment to even consider quitting, because there was always another therapy to try. Besides, I knew my mother wasn't going to stop until I was better. My years of vigorous training enabled me to keep moving. I just kept taking steps forward, unsure of where they would lead.

*I was flipping through **People** magazine one April morning in 1994 when I came across an article about a Dr. Bernard Brucker, working out of Jackson Memorial Hospital in Miami, Florida. Dr. Brucker had discovered that the brain, brain stem, and spinal cord have many extra cells that aren't used during our typical lifespan.*

Under the right conditions, those extra cells can be awakened and utilized to re-place damaged cells. I don't remember much of the article, but one particular quote of Dr. Brucker's stuck with me: "You bring me someone with one brain cell, and I will rebuild their body and awaken other brain cells."

I immediately called Dr. Brucker's office to set up an appointment. When we arrived, Dr. Brucker informed us that each of Jennifer's appointments would be exactly fifty minutes long, and that if we arrived five minutes late, then her ap-pointment would be shortened to forty-five minutes long. Jennifer and I just looked at each other. We knew we would never be late.

With no other formalities, Dr. Brucker assessed Jennifer. After watching her walk, he announced that she was walking flat-footed and that she needed to develop a "heel strike." He swept us off into the therapy room, where there was a large video screen on the wall and a computer technician at a desk. The doctor and the tech put sensors on certain muscles in her legs, and then asked her to take a step.

Two graph-like vertical lines, running against two horizontal lines about twelve inches apart, appeared on the big screen. "Now, Jennifer," Dr. Brucker said. "Next time you take a step, think of keeping those vertical lines in between the two hori-zontal lines."

Amazingly, in the next couple of steps, she managed to do it. Her muscle move-ment was represented by those vertical lines, and the goal was always to keep the vertical lines in between the horizontal ones. When she saw the results on the monitor, her brain would then process the information and learn from this tech-nique, which we later found out was called biofeedback. By focusing on the verti-cal lines and striving to keep them between the horizontal lines, which gradually moved closer and closer together, Jen was training her brain and body to refine her physical movements. Each step she took allowed her brain to use the new in-formation and retrain her muscles.

By the time we left that day, the horizontal lines were an inch apart, and she was able to keep the vertical lines within those boundaries. At the end of the ses-sion, when Jennifer was unhooked from the sensors, she was able to walk with a normal gait—utilizing a heel strike for the very first time since her accident.

As I met Dr. Brucker's gaze, no words were needed. "You can't do it," he said.

"But why not?" I asked.

"You cannot come in every day until you've rebuilt her from the ground up. The brain can't take it. But because Jennifer is young and strong, we will go as far as we can. When we see her brain getting tired, we'll take a break, and come back to it later."

He was right. We had to pace ourselves and take a weeklong break after every two weeks. So we drove four hours round-trip every day from our Florida house to Miami for our fifty-minute appointment. During the long drive, I would make Jennifer read the story of Chicken Little out loud to me from a Little Golden Book (which she hated). I also made her sing along repeatedly with "Can You Feel The Love Tonight," from **The Lion King**. The message of the song had nothing to do with me making her sing it; I just wanted Jennifer to gain voice projection, breath, and intonation. After thousands of miles logged on I-95, I watched my daughter begin to regain control of her body. And we were never late.

Alice Quaid, craniosacral therapist

First, to explain what craniosacral therapy is, remember Silly Putty? And how, when you pull too quickly or too hard, Silly Putty rips apart? But when you pull it gently, it stretches and stretches? That helps describe how I wanted to help open up Jennifer's craniosacral system to allow as much recovery to occur as possible through brain plasticity. Through gentle pulling, I wanted to get all the stretching that might be available for her.

When I met the Fields at the Upledger Institute, I found them fascinating. They were combining alternative medicine with traditional medicine back when no one else was doing that. Jennifer found me "very traditional." But although I worked at Upledger, which was not the most traditional medical location, my training as an osteopath allowed me to understand the extent of damage her brain had suffered. The difference between where she was right after the accident and where she is today is, for lack of a better word, a miracle. But in between there was a *lot* of hard work.

Jen's system was compressed; the flow of her cerebrospinal fluid was impeded. I believed getting more cranial movement would increase her brain's ability to use its plasticity and thereby improve its ability to heal by shifting workloads from injured to healthy areas. I also felt more cranial movement

---

would allow Jen to gain increased cognitive function, again through the brain's increased plasticity.

Craniosacral therapy was first developed in the 1930s by William Sutherland, an osteopath, and involves light touches on the head. Sutherland believed that body manipulation was a better method of healing than using drugs. Sutherland felt the body has its own healing capacity that could be facilitated by kneading the soft tissues, as in massage. Sutherland also saw that the body has cyclic energies that flow in mid-tides and long tides.

Therapists using approaches like massage and craniosacral work always noticed that bodywork brought out emotions. Back in the 1980s, researcher Candace Pert theorized that emotion peptides existed in the brain's lymph system and moved from the brain to the body letting the emotions rise during and after bodywork. Little hard evidence existed for this theory until the spring of 2015, when the discovery of a lymph system in the brain showed evidence of links and pathways to the body's lymph system. The two systems are now considered one.

Craniosacral work helped Jen's other therapies be more effective: physical therapy and Brainwave Technology therapy, for example. In particular, Jen's progress with Continuum was strongly aided by my work on her. The domino effect of craniosacral work on other therapies shows that Jen and Joanne found the right therapy at the right time. I admire Joanne's energy and all the work she did networking and struggling to find practitioners. Her efforts enabled the Fields to make a new, innovative blend of alternative medicine with traditional medicine. They were far ahead of their time!

Chapter 9

A Window to the World

We were so fortunate to have so many smart, genuinely kind people in our lives to help Jennifer in her recovery. People were always surprising us, making huge differences, sometimes without even being aware of it.

After Jen's accident, there was a period of time where she struggled with her vision. I didn't realize this. Her right eye had opened fully as a result of Martha's therapies, and I assumed everything was fine until someone asked me offhandedly if Jen had had her eyes checked recently, and I realized she hadn't. They went on to tell me that, because of Jen's head injury, her eyes might be sending her brain the wrong signals, causing her to move her body incorrectly. I was stunned to think we might have missed a necessary and important step in Jen's recovery. I began devoting myself to finding the best eye specialist for traumatic brain injury.

We found a world-renowned behavioral optometrist, Dr. William Padula, at the Padula Institute of Vision in Guilford, Connecticut. His research had proven that visual problems associated with head injuries often interfere with balance and coordination because your body responds instinctively to whatever you see.

Dr. Padula told us that after a head injury, the eyes often don't translate what they see in the way they once did. It was only then that we realized I was seeing things at an angle and unconsciously trying to make my body fit into the distorted space. To help retrain my eyes, Dr. Padula gave me glasses with adjustable yoked prisms. Almost immediately, my body adjusted to the fact that I was finally seeing my surroundings normally. My shoulders straightened and my gait evened out. We were amazed that this seemingly tiny change could make such a big difference.

I had heard over and over again from various physical therapists, "Jennifer, drop your left hip and raise your right shoulder." She could do it for a few minutes with total concentration but then she would slip back into her "normal" way of walking. Now all of a sudden, with one pair of glasses, she straightened up and walked smoothly down the hall. She clearly felt the change, too, and she turned around and beamed at me.

William V. Padula, OD, FAAO, FNORA, DPNAP, neuro-optometrist and founder of the Padula Institute of Vision

When Jennifer first came to me as a patient, she struggled with posture, balance, movement, speech, and vision. After evaluating her, I found that her visual problems were related to dysfunction in the spatial-visual process, which, in turn, affected her balance and posture.

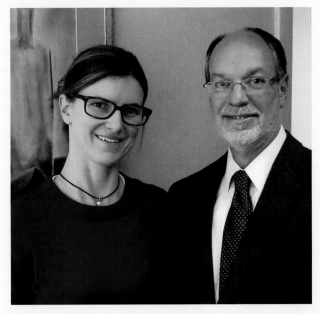

With Dr. Padula

It was clear that Jennifer was struggling, trying to fight her way back from a devastating injury. As I worked with her, I quickly learned that she was not the type of person to just give up. She accepted her injuries, but she was a fighter through and through. I learned about her history as a world-class equestrian, and it became clear that the competitor in Jennifer was ready to rise to the occasion—only this time, she was fighting her way back to her sense of self, to increased intent and independence, and to a quality of life that she wanted.

One of the first things I did was prescribe special prism lenses to help influence the spatial-visual process—the basis of our eyesight, the platform on which we begin to think and process details. A general eye doctor typically focuses on the higher-level system—what you see and how you see it—with little regard to that basis. Jennifer had post-trauma vision syndrome (PTVS)—a complete collapse of the spatial-visual process. PTVS causes patients to see the world as a mass of details, an experience akin to driving in a snowstorm with your high beams on: there's a barrage of snowflakes coming at you and you can see each one but not the road beyond. To someone with PTVS, the world gets overwhelming very, very quickly; they can't deal with any movement in their peripheral vision because everything appears in stark detail, like the flakes in that snowstorm. Being in a grocery store or in a busy environment can be shocking.

The prism glasses I prescribed for Jennifer were designed to balance her spatial-visual process, and to treat another condition she had called, visual midline syndrome (VMS). With VMS, the entire concept of centering the body based on the visual system is distorted and this was influencing Jennifer's balance.

We used a variety of treatments to address Jen's issues, and with improvement in vision came improvement in cognition, balance, speech, and language. She continues to make great progress, and I'm very pleased. Not all patients have the tenacity to stay with therapy; many think you can make only a limited amount of progress in a finite amount of time, but that's not the case and Jennifer proves it. She's continued to improve physically, to maintain social relationships, and to live a meaningful life. Jennifer is one of those extraordinary persons with the motivation and the means to continue her healing process. She's not only a fighter, but one of the happiest persons with whom I have had the opportunity to work.

The glasses helped with my balance and even woke up my right eye, which I hadn't been able to see out of clearly since my accident. Unfortunately, once my right eye became functional I started seeing double. Dr. Padula gave me several visual exercises to work on, and years later he decided that I should wear prism glasses over contact lenses to correct my depth perception and widen my window of vision. I have also had surgery to try to lessen my double vision. Now I have about a fourteen-inch window of single vision; beyond it I have double vision. To this day, my eyes don't always work together perfectly. But I continue to work hard, and I see Dr. Padula throughout the year. My vision is a work in progress.

On one of our visits to see Dr. Padula, I asked him if he had any other thoughts about therapists we should see. He recommended a physical therapist, Dr. Christine Nelson, whom he knew quite well. A licensed physical therapist from Johns Hopkins University, Dr. Nelson had gone to Cuernavaca, Mexico, to help a friend work with underprivileged children with brain injuries. She liked the area so much—and the medical freedom that it afforded—that she decided to stay and open a clinic there.

Around the same time, my mother happened to be in Mexico with the World Wildlife Fund to watch the migration of the monarch butterflies. She agreed to make a side trip out to the clinic to meet Dr. Nelson. She reported back that I needed to take Jen to meet Dr. Nelson personally. She knew I would be apprehensive about traveling to Mexico, but she felt there was something about Dr. Nelson that was worth further exploration. (She had a sixth sense about such things.)

My mother agreed to meet us in Mexico City; I'll never forget seeing her on the other side of the customs checkpoint waiting when our plane landed. Estaban, the clinic's driver, met us at the airport and drove us the two hours to the air-conditioned hotel I'd found for us just outside of Cuernavaca, in the neighboring town of Sumia.

When we got to the clinic the next day, we found it was very clean and each wall was painted a traditional Mexican color: red, deep blue, rich grass green, and golden yellow. It seemed a happy and cheerful environment, but that contrasted drastically with our reception. No one would speak to us. We sat on a bench while people walked by us as if we were invisible. We had come all this way and made all this effort and we had no idea why we were being ignored. Finally, I asked the desk what was going on. It seems there had been some miscommunication, and they had booked us a reservation at their local hotel, which of course had gone unused. It was not exactly the best start to our time with a woman who would turn out to be one of our best therapists.

Once everything was worked out with the hotels, we went in for our first session. Appointments were divided into three parts: first, Jennifer would have a hands-on session with Dr. Nelson, then she would have vision therapy, and last, she would work with a physical and occupational therapist.

Because we had a lot of free time when we weren't at the clinic, we wanted to visit various sites around the countryside that Dr. Nelson had recommended. I didn't speak any Spanish and we had a hard time getting around. I asked the desk clerk several times to find us a cab driver who spoke English. "No problem!" he would *answer with a big grin. The next morning we would happily get in our taxi, I would say, "Please take us to the clinic," and the driver would look at me wide-eyed and answer, "No speak English." After this had happened a multitude of times, I finally found a wonderful cab driver named Gonzalo, who did speak English. He remained our driver for the duration of our trip and became our friend.*

One day, we went to see an Indian outpost called Tepoztlán, where there were many wonderful displays by local artists offering colorful pottery for sale. Jennifer became obsessed with the pottery and would make her way through the vendors, constantly bartering with the locals. I don't know if it was the bright colors of the pottery that attracted her, but she was obsessed. She disappeared once, and we ran frantically up and down the rows of vendors until we finally found her in a small booth, leaning over the pots. She was repeating the price she was willing to pay in pesos, and the old Mexican man in the booth was shaking his head. Finally, they came to an agreement and she walked away with her treasure for the day and a big smile. This experience represented freedom and, more importantly, normalcy for her. The locals responded to her and didn't act as if there was anything wrong. In a sense, Jennifer liked the competition of the bartering and so did the vendors. Needless to say, we ended up with more than a few boxes of pottery to take back to the States with us!

I remember as we walked towards the outpost, my eyes began to widen. I had never seen anything like it! I was fascinated by all of the bright, colorful pieces of pottery in different shapes. I walked down the aisles followed by my mother and Mike. My eyes were drawn in many different directions and I wanted every single clay animal and pot. I felt like my own person again as I started haggling with the local sellers, and I felt a rush of adrenalin as I got them to lower the price of each piece. I don't think Mom and Mike shared my enthusiasm as the bags of pottery multiplied.

We went back to Dr. Nelson's clinic twice a year for the next few years. Each time we went, we'd stay for two weeks (and inevitably buy more pottery). On one trip, I mentioned Jennifer's right arm to Dr. Nelson—Christine to us now—and she examined it. The arm had never been fully straightened by the Dynasplint and never integrated into her full body movement. Jen used it, but overcompensated with her left arm even though she was right-handed. And, when she stood up, her right arm bent to a ninety-degree angle.

Mike Martin, Fields' property caretaker and friend

The trips to Cuernavaca, Mexico, were some that I will never forget. At that time, Mrs. Field was following a strict diet, eating the exact same foods every day: baguettes from our local bakery with local butter and fresh mozzarella, plus OJ and grapefruit juice. So I got on the plane to Mexico with suitcases filled with food! Who goes cross-country with suitcases filled with food? I had twenty warm loaves of bread in my carry-on; the whole plane smelled like a bakery! When I arrived, we had to cram all the butter and cheese into the hotel room's tiny refrigerator.

Christine Nelson was a genius and every time we went Jennifer would show huge improvement. When we were not at the clinic, we always went on some outing with our cabdriver, Gonzalo. (Mrs. Field finally found a driver that really did speak English.) We went to Taxco, a small town on the top of a hill where every store, it seemed, sold silver for very cheap prices. We were big customers. We went to Tepoztlán where Jen bartered wih the Mexican Indians for their brightly painted pottery. I began to wonder, as it piled up in the hotel if we'd get it home or if Jen would open a store!

Jen still had a sporadic tremor in her left arm when we were in Cuernavaca. At lunch she would spontaneously fling her food and it would fly at me because I sat to her right. We'd laugh and laugh. It never missed me! We shared another laugh when Jen took a liking to a waiter at our hotel. He styled his hair up into a point, and Mrs. Field nicknamed him the "tufted titmouse." Jen would go out of her way to drag me to breakfast, the pool, or wherever he was. She couldn't be on her own, so that became my new job.

One night when we drove to a nearby restaurant in the rain, we were almost washed away by a flash flood that came roaring down the hill and up to the sides of the taxi. "Don't worry, we'll be fine," Gonzalo said. We were terrified but we really were fine, and Gonzalo chuckled all the way back to the hotel.

There we were, the three of us, on another adventure where we were able to watch Jennifer make huge strides forward. I began to see a real future for her.

"Hmmm. Interesting," said Christine, gripping Jen's arm. "Well, sometimes you just have to do . . . **this***."*

I heard a "crack" as Christine snapped Jen's arm forcefully. Shocked, I expected to hear Jennifer scream in pain but she was in no pain at all and, magically it seemed, could move her arm back and forth normally again. I just sat there marveling at Christine's ingenuity and guts, which influenced every therapy at her clinic.

I had a tremor in my left hand, and Dr. Nelson's therapy involved using two pencils with erasers, one held in each hand. My task was to stack small dice using the erasers. When I asked how I could possibly do this with my tremor, Dr. Nelson told me that when the brain uses both hands together to do a task, it usually overrides a tremor . . . and she was right! I successfully stacked those dice with the pencil erasers, one on top of the other. I was amazed!

I loved to go to Cuernavaca because the energy of the clinic was so positive. The therapists who worked with me were relatively young, and they made the tasks at hand fun—which, in turn, made me look forward to my sessions. Dr. Nelson's clinic offered a variety of different therapies, some of which my Mom tried too. On one trip Mike agreed to attend his own session to try to treat his severe migraines. A therapist named Doreen used her elbows to squeeze his head in different places, and now? No more migraines—not since therapy at Dr. Nelson's clinic.

Christine Nelson was a genius, and we were so fortunate to cross paths with her when we did. I recommended Dr. Nelson to many families that I met along the way. One woman called me a week after her son with severe brain damage had started therapy there, and she told me that Dr. Nelson had made more progress with her son in that one week than all the other centers they'd been to had in three years. I was thrilled!

Not too long after this phone call, that same woman called my mother again. She broke the terribly sad news that Dr. Nelson had died suddenly. Mom and I were heartbroken. We counted Dr. Nelson as one of our friends and saviors ever since our very first trip to the clinic. The world of traumatic brain injury lost one of its greatest innovators and therapists that day.

Over a year after my accident, I drove with my mother and grandmother to the Omega Institute in Rhinebeck, New York. My mother, through her long hours of

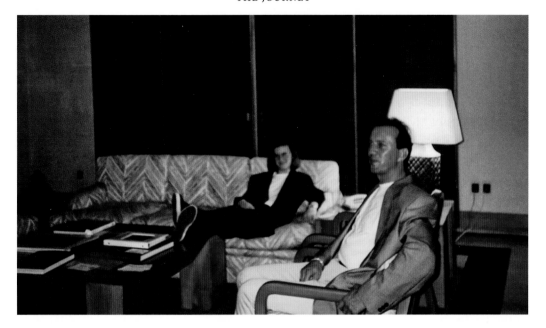

In Cuernavaca with Mike Martin

research into different therapies, had learned about a woman named Emilie Conrad who was giving a workshop on her therapy, Continuum Movement.

Anyone who knew us back then knew that the Omega Institute, where Emilie Conrad was holding her workshop, would be just about the last place on the planet that we would drive to on a beautiful fall day. I pictured us being greeted by a bunch of people wearing Birkenstocks and munching on granola. As a matter of fact, I had recently heard a story about a class being offered at the Institute on self-love, the only requirement for which was to bring a hand-held mirror. I didn't ask any questions. But I'd read that Emilie's work was beneficial to nerve regeneration and strengthening soft tissue, so we were willing to brave the Birkenstocks and leave our comfort zone once again.

Emilie agreed to see me during the lunch break of her workshop that day. I remember a long walk across an uneven grassy area; the distance might have been only fifty feet, but I still had problems walking. I was excited and nervous at the same time. We had no idea where on the campus to go to find Emilie, so we just started opening doors. Behind the first door we opened, drums were beating loudly, which was a little off-putting as, since my head injury, loud noises and I did not mix well. By the time we found someone to ask for directions and found Emilie, I was exhausted.

Emilie Conrad was a forceful, grounded woman with very dark hair. She had an ageless beauty. My overwhelming feeling upon meeting her was that whatever she was doing, I wanted to do it too. She talked with us about Jennifer's history and the possible role of Continuum in her recovery. She also explained how she had cured herself of a life-threatening disease in her twenties, using movement and breath in a way that would become her creation, Continuum Movement.

After a bit of introduction, Emilie had me lay down on my back on the floor, and she lay down next to me. She then asked me to raise my right arm—the one I'd been having so much trouble with—off of the floor as slowly as I could. She explained that incredibly slow "micro-movements" could awaken the nerves and their connections to the brain. It took me about half an hour, under Emilie's direction, to raise and lower my right arm. By the time I had finished, my arm felt light as a feather, but I was exhausted. She explained that this was the work I had to do to retrain my arm's motion.

Emilie specifically told us that she wanted Jennifer to take between ten and twenty minutes to raise her right arm a foot or so off the ground, and then take the same amount of time to bring it down. It was as difficult to watch as it was for Jennifer to do it. I was intrigued, but secretly wondered if the visit had been worth the long drive. In retrospect, I realize how sometimes the smallest things can make the biggest differences, and that the most marvelous things can be found in the strangest places. In later years, I followed the Omega Institute and learned about all of the amazing people who pass through their doors.

When we went home, Jennifer incorporated Emilie's teachings into her rehabilitation, and she found that she could truly feel a difference. The Continuum movements were much more powerful than they initially appeared. Over the next few years, Jennifer traveled to many of Emilie's workshops, and she benefitted greatly. Continuum Movement proved to be one of the most successful therapies in her recovery process.

Continuum Movement uses Emilie's theory of the body as a fluid organism in combination with breath, sound, and movement to help retrain the body to move in slower and more fluid ways. After years of practicing it, I can close my eyes and go to a place in my brain where I am so much more physically agile, which in itself is incredibly freeing because I'm not trapped by any physical limitations. I continue to practice Continuum today, and I'm still discovering new ways of moving.

Emilie Conrad, founder of Continuum Movement

When I first saw Jen, I felt she was in an extreme state of suspension. She had suffered an extreme degree of shock and been in a coma for two months following her accident. I felt that the coma was still evident in her body, but Jennifer's spirit was not ready to cash in. Her championship nature added to her determination to succeed. Jennifer was used to going for the gold. She was used to training and she was used to being challenged. I would like to take a lot of the credit for her recovery, but I must say she has an indomitable spirit.

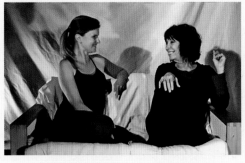

Jennifer and Emilie Conrad

My theory is that the fluid in the body, the fluid in the planet, and the fluid in the galaxy represent one stream of what I call "biocosmic intelligence." This belief is the basis of Continuum. Jen was a fabulous candidate for this work because of her champion tendencies. When I said, "You need to practice this for at least an hour or two every day," she replied, "Is that all?"

Chapter 10

STALLED OUT AND RESTARTED

IN THE BEGINNING OF MY JOURNEY TO RECOVERY, I never really got depressed. But as I improved and I became more aware of the challenges I faced, depression crept in at times. I fretted that I wasn't responding to therapies fast enough. Or that maybe we had stalled out. We needed to find something else.

In the fall of 1994, Dr. Grassi, Jennifer's pediatrician for many years, invited me to Crotched Mountain Rehabilitation Center to meet with their therapists and share some of what I'd learned during my travels with Jen. The hope was that some of what we had discovered would help in treating some of their patients. Yet as I sat at the large table with all of the therapists, I realized they were highly skeptical about many of the less conventional therapies we had explored over the past two years. Their skepticism didn't diminish my belief in the benefits of what we were doing. So I forged on, and told them about everything that had benefitted Jennifer.

At the end of the meeting, one of them offhandedly tossed a brochure across the table at me and said, "Here, you might be interested in this." The brochure, entitled **Whispers from the Brain**, outlined the research and theories of Dr. Margaret Ayers. Dr. Ayers was a pioneer in neurofeedback, a technique similar to biofeedback that she believed could retrain the brain.

I couldn't drive down that mountain fast enough to begin learning more. I burst through the door and told Jennifer, "I think I've found our next therapy! It's called neurofeedback." From reading the pamphlet carefully, I learned about a woman named Janet Bloom who had worked with Dr. Ayers for two years. To my surprise she was living in nearby Hopkinton, New Hampshire. Janet Bloom was one of the very few people to study directly under Dr. Ayers, and we were able to see her for several sessions. After each session, Jennifer seemed much brighter and more with it.

When I mentioned we were planning to travel to Los Angeles again, Janet very generously suggested going to see Dr. Ayers in person. Dr. Ayers met with Jennifer, talked to her about her traumatic brain injury, sat her down in front of a *computer, and hooked two sensors up to Jen's scalp, each monitoring a different part of her brain. The computer screen showed her brainwaves on one side and, on the other side, a tube with a blue line across its middle with a bubble inside. The computer program allowed the brain to control the bubble on a subconscious level. The goal was for Jen to keep the bubble under the line by using her thought processes (similar, again, to the biofeedback with Dr. Brucker).*

In the beginning, the bubble went above the line, but as Jennifer worked with the program, she was able to build back the connection between her brain and her nervous system and keep the bubble below the line. Jennifer loved the challenge of finding the right mental balance to keep the bubble low. It was a totally competitive event for her, and it was the perfect kind of therapy for her personality. We both felt that neurofeedback was invaluable, and we stuck with it for many years.

At one appointment with Dr. Ayers, we asked her about finding a new nutritionist, and she directed us to Dr. Tobin Watkinson in Santa Monica. She told us we might like him because he was "normal" and very bright. My mom called and luckily they had had a cancellation for that afternoon. Like many facets of my recovery, it seemed fated.

Dr. Watkinson is a physicist, a biochemist, a chiropractor, and a naturopath. He is also a medical intuitive, which means he can diagnose you from looking at a picture or from talking to you on the phone. During our appointment that afternoon, he used kinesiology (muscle testing) at certain acupuncture points to determine his course of treatment.

Most of Dr. Watkinson's treatment revolves around his method of testing, homeopathy, and nutrition. Over the years he has worked with me on both the physical and mental levels, which has been a huge help. He has also been able to comfortably integrate appropriate nutrients, supplements, and vitamins into my lifestyle. I still see him in person two to three times a year. We have worked together now for more than fifteen years and he has filled in a huge piece in my recovery puzzle.

Janet Bloom, psycho-neuro physiologist

I was trained by Dr. Margaret Ayers to perform digital, real-time neurofeedback. This therapy teaches patients like Jennifer to use a high-speed computer to retrain their brainwaves. Neurofeedback, also known as "electroencephalograph (EEG) biofeedback," differs from standard biofeedback, which only trains patients to control elements of their autonomic nervous system, like their blood pressure and heart rate.

The brain has no feedback mechanism to fix itself or see its own damage. The underlying premise of computerized feedback is to provide the patient with a way to see the damage and fix it over time. Using electrodes, neurofeedback creates a brain map for therapy.

Dr. Ayers treated clients from all over the world at her Beverly Hills' practice, Neuropathways EEG Imaging. When she began in the 1970s, long before the development of sophisticated software programs, she hired an engineer to build custom computer hardware to accommodate her therapy protocol, which required the placement of ten to twenty electrodes in standardized systems or patterns, according to the patient's disability.

Jen's severe TBI coupled with her long coma affected a lot of her functioning. She really fought to gain more. For example, patients with TBI often struggle to stay awake and remain conscious and alert, and Jennifer had a hard time staying awake. Over a couple months of treatment at my practice in New Hampshire, her affect changed to being bright and more wide-awake.

You have to work gently with damaged brains, so Jen could only have one half-hour weekly session. It took two or three years for her to regain stamina, a more fluid gait, and better vision. I worked with her throughout her years at Wheaton College, and then over the next twelve years for maintenance sessions.

Jennifer and Joanne are incredible humans. I've seen many pairs like them—an extremely dynamic parent shepherding an injured child. It's breathtaking when their struggle ends in triumph, as the Fields' has. I've learned so much from those dynamic, incredible parents!

D. Tobin Watkinson, DC, director of the Tobin Institute, Inc., and specialist in patient-centered alternative and complementary healthcare

My first patient for the day was one I had never met. I had very little background on her—a phone call from her mother to schedule the appointment was all. I opened the door to my waiting room and there was Jen: a beautiful young lady whose movements, even at first glance, indicated that something major had happened to her. Her speech was slow and she stopped frequently mid-sentence to gather her thoughts. She was clear about one thing, though: she was determined to get well and to do anything and everything to accomplish this goal.

That first appointment, nearly fifteen years ago, followed a very delicate eye surgery. Although the operation had been successful, Jennifer's eyes did not track together and, as she explained it, her vision was "broken." Images were fractured or split, making the simplest tasks nearly impossible. She walked like a drunken sailor, bouncing from wall to wall.

Proprioception is the unconscious perception of movement and spatial orientation that arises from body stimuli. The brain takes cues from hearing, sight, and the balance mechanism in your ears, and integrates that information with the proprioceptive mechanisms of the joints. I realized that I had to engage the rest of Jennifer's body to reintegrate her vision back into rhythm with her eyes via the joints of her body. I started to work immediately, tapping away on every deep tendon reflex. I began with her upper extremities, then moved to her lower ones. One joint after another, I tapped away until I got a consistent reflex. After each reintegration I would have her walk, and with each one her walking got better.

Our list of goals was quite long. Some days, we would work from sun up until nearly midnight, and I remember several times working for days on end. We worked on her body's electrical system to integrate her own electronics; we worked on her nutrition to help pathways of inflammation, detoxification, and allergies all function to their maximum. Her muscles and coordination were of major importance early on, and we developed at least one technique that I have since been able to use on hundreds of other patients to integrate injuries and restore function.

Jennifer never tired, she never said, "Enough!" She had a goal, and nothing was going to get in the way of success. That was the Jennifer we all came to know, as we became part of her healing and part of her goal.

"Rome"

Rome
sitting at a café
the sun beating down
a droplet of perspiration cascading down my forehead
life
people walking on a slow journey
where?
all the colors fading as the sun goes down
vitality diminishing
the ochre staying in my mind
the hope that vitality might stay within surrounding me
everything crumbles
crumbles

—Jennifer

Part III

A Brave New World

When I was seventeen, they said I would go to the Olympics.
I didn't.
I went so much further.

Chapter 11

College Years

MOST OF MY FRIENDS WENT OFF TO COLLEGE when they graduated from high school, but because of my accident I thought it would be impossible for me. After two years of constant rehabilitation, however, I decided that maybe I could do it. I wanted to go to college; to be, in my mind, "normal," but it was crucial that I keep up with the recovery process. Therapy was what I did, day in and day out. Every day at home I would work on my own. At times it was hard for me to know if I was completing the exercises as they were prescribed, and Mike would come over to help me do them correctly. My whole life centered around exercises and finding new treatments, new therapies, and new doctors. But I was nineteen, and I wanted something more.

I started to have visions of being a student again. To get myself back in the swing of things, I decided to enroll in a math class at The Dublin School. I failed miserably. Undaunted, I refocused my energies and took a writing class at Keene State College, twenty miles away. I was thrilled to get an A in the class. I'd always excelled in math and science prior to the accident, but at this point those subjects were beyond me. It didn't matter. I had a story to tell.

In 1995, I told my mom that it was time for me to go away to college. I knew she wanted me to have more recovery under my belt before I left, but I felt ready. Looking back, I realize it wasn't just college courses I needed—it was the social life that being on campus would bring, too. I went to meet with a college advisor who knew of only one school that might be accepting of my situation. That school was Wheaton College in Norton, Massachusetts, and so I applied.

At that time, Wheaton didn't require SAT scores but they did ask for further testing to see if I was capable of completing the coursework. We found someone in Connecticut to administer the tests, and the results were mixed. In some categories I tested at a second grade level—but at others, I performed at graduate school level. It didn't matter to me what the tests said. This was something I had to do even though I knew it would be a stretch.

About four months after I applied to Wheaton, I was down in the barn with Swanny. I looked up suddenly, and I saw my mother running toward the barn in her pink bathrobe, frantically waving an envelope above her head. I knew immediately what it was. She handed me the envelope, which she had already opened. I could tell by the look on her face that the news was good. I read the first few words of the letter, "We are pleased to inform you. . . ." I looked at my mother who hugged me and burst into tears. I was stunned and excited . . . and panicked! I'd been completely closeted for the last three years with just my mom, my family, Mike, and therapists to interact with. Suddenly I was heading out into a whole new world alone!

Before I left for college, I was able to visit my half-brother, Peter, who was living in Rome at the time. It was my first trip abroad alone. (It was my first trip *anywhere* alone, and of course I couldn't just stay in the same country!) My mother was practically apoplectic with worry. Her only consolation came from the fact that Peter had a friend with Italian government clearance that allowed him to meet me right at the gate.

Peter, who was teaching European history at an American school at the time, was the perfect older brother, and a fantastic host. He took good care of me, and in the Italian way, we savored our days. We went sightseeing in the mornings, then ate lunch and napped in the afternoons. It was a great pace for me, and I fell in love with the city. It was the reason I planned to study Italian at Wheaton—I could picture making a life for myself in Rome.

Life is amazing. Three years after my accident, I was in Rome, and then suddenly, I was at college, unpacking my bags and enlisting other students to help me drag furniture into my dorm. I had a great roommate, Nathalie, from Haiti. I was taking all kinds of classes. I kept thinking to myself, *I was just sleeping in a hospital bed with orderlies passing by, and now I'm a freshman in college. I just learned how to speak English again, and now I'm taking an Italian class!* I was beginning a new phase of my recovery—a phase that did not constantly involve doctors, healers, or nutritionists, although I did continue my therapies during breaks and sometimes on weekends. Yet as I watched my mom drive away, all of a sudden, I got very sad. It was the first time in my life that I was living without her, but I was determined to do it.

I had gotten permission from Wheaton to take only three courses a semester. One course was a poetry class, and I realized very quickly that writing poetry was an

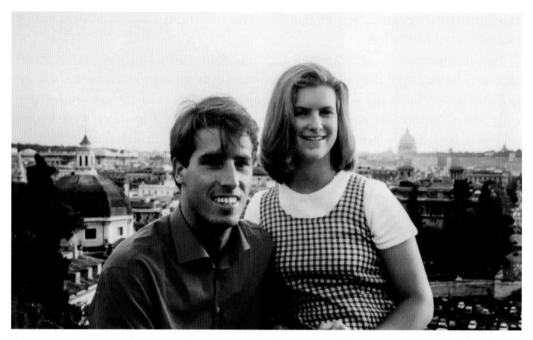

In Rome, with brother, Peter Miller

effective way for me to wade in and sort through all of the emotions that I needed to deal with. My incredible professor, Pozzi Escot, was able to coach me in my writing, and entered one of my poems into the National Poetry Society contest. My poem, "Rome," was accepted. I was a freshman in college, and I had a published poem!

Two or three weeks into my freshman year, I went to a party. I knew I shouldn't drink, but I wanted to fit in so I had two shots of gin. For someone who hadn't consumed alcohol in two years and who had a brain injury, two shots of gin was a lot. The alcohol hit me quickly, and I became instantly drunk. Someone—I don't remember who—helped me back to my room, where I tripped over Nathalie's bed and fell on the floor. I managed to crawl into my own bed without waking her up. When I woke up hung-over and bleary-eyed the next morning, my first thought was, "*Wow. My thumb really hurts.*"

After a trip to the local infirmary where I was told my thumb was just bruised, not broken, I reluctantly called my mother. I was reluctant because I didn't want to disappoint her and, frankly, because I was a little afraid of what I had done to my thumb. She had been supportive of me going to school, but she had also been un-derstandably apprehensive because she was afraid something would happen when she wasn't there to take care of it (I'd had nightmares of her moving in with Nathalie and me to ensure my safety).

I also did not want to tell her that I'd been drunk. I was embarrassed, so I just told a little white lie and said that I had slammed my thumb in a door. My mother, of course, was smart enough to know that I had *not* just slammed my thumb in a door and eventually the truth came out.

When Jennifer went to college, all my friends and family wondered how I would carry on without my daughter at my side. For almost three years, we had been joined at the hip, struggling through this traumatic event together. The truth of the matter was, I was really ready to have some time to myself. When Jen called about her thumb, I was knee-deep in my closet, sorting and organizing my clothes. The news of her injured thumb flipped me out completely, and I almost just told her to deal with it herself. However, duty called, and I contacted Massachusetts General Hospital.

Because my mother can do anything she sets her mind to, she somehow got an appointment on very short notice with a leading hand surgeon, Dr. Jesse Jupiter. I made the trip to Mass General Hospital, and he told me I'd fractured my thumb. If the break had been a millimeter longer, I would have had to have surgery and wear a cast for six months. I thanked a higher power for small favors. As it was, I had to wear a brace on my right hand, so now I had to try to take notes with my left hand, tremor and all. Not really a good start to my college experience, given all my other disabilities.

You'd think I would have quit drinking, but it wasn't until I did neurofeedback again with Janet Bloom that I really stopped. She told me about the detrimental effects that alcohol has on the brain and how it negates neurofeedback. I realized I simply couldn't keep adding that complication to my body, which I'd been trying so hard to take care of.

During the summer after my sophomore year, I went to Florida to do hyperbaric oxygen therapy, which isolates the patient in a pressure chamber to deliver more oxygen to the brain. My mom had heard of many beneficial results for people with head injuries. She had heard that hyperbaric oxygen treatment could awaken brain cells that had been dormant since an accident or stroke. I hoped this could really help me.

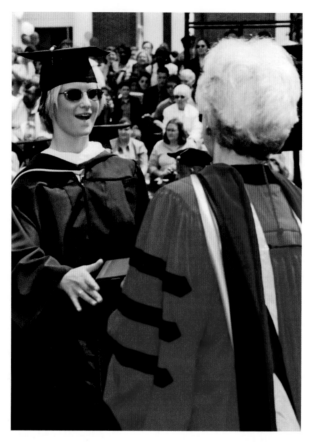

Receiving her diploma from Wheaton's president, Dale Rogers Marshall

When they first put Jennifer in the hyperbaric chamber and closed the lid, it took all my strength not to run in and yank the lid open. The chamber was so small it reminded me of an MRI tube, and it scared me. I didn't want to lock my daughter in that tiny space. As usual, though, I hung in there and hoped for a great result. There were other people in the waiting room, so I tried to reassure myself by engaging them in conversation about the treatment. Most of the feedback was positive, and I started to feel a bit better.

Almost immediately following the treatment, I noticed that Jen's impulses seemed more controlled. Since her accident, if anyone mentioned needing to, say, hail a taxi, she would have run into the middle of the street to try to stop one. The fact that she seemed more levelheaded was really encouraging. The speed *of her speech also improved, as did her intonation. After two weeks, though, she complained of dizziness and a headache, so we stopped the hyperbaric oxygen treatments. It was really hard to just quit because of all of the improvements she'd made, but the pain in her head was so pronounced that we had no other choice.*

By the time summer rolled around, the pain in my head was constant, sometimes getting worse and never going away. Aspirin, Aleve, Advil . . . nothing worked. I flew out to California to work with Margaret Ayers again in the hope she could solve the problem. Unfortunately, neurofeedback didn't fix it. Burdened by the constant pain, I was forced to take the year off from college. During that year we consulted specialists at UCLA and Johns Hopkins. Unfortunately, they couldn't come up with an answer; they attributed the pain to my brain injury. To this day, I'm still affected by this problem that we have yet to solve.

When I returned to school as a junior in 1998, the rest of my class was in their final year. It was very weird for me, but I pretended I was a senior myself, spending time with all my classmates whenever I could and attending senior events at the end of the year.

During the second semester of my sophomore year at Wheaton, I had taken an art history class. I had always wanted to take the class, but everyone had said there was too much memorization, and I'd been afraid to attempt it. Now, though, I was ready to take the plunge. I ended up falling completely in love with the subject and the professors, and by the middle of that year, I declared art history as my major.

"How can you study art history? There's so much memorization!" people kept asking me. Like a lot of other things in my life, though, once I'd found something that seemed to fit me so well I was determined to make it work. I loved art history so much that it didn't matter how much hard work would be needed. I knew I had the discipline.

None of it would have been possible without the help and guidance of my advisor and art history professor, Evelyn Staudinger. She has since become a lifelong friend. I will always look up to her and be grateful for everything she did. I clearly remember taking one of her exams for a gothic art class. The allotted two hours passed, and every single one of the other students had long since completed the exam and left. Not me, though. Wheaton runs on an honor system, so Professor Staudinger told me, "Just leave the exam under my door when you're done."

I was incredibly fortunate to have supportive professors at Wheaton. With that kind of support, I couldn't possibly let anyone at the school down. Wheaton didn't

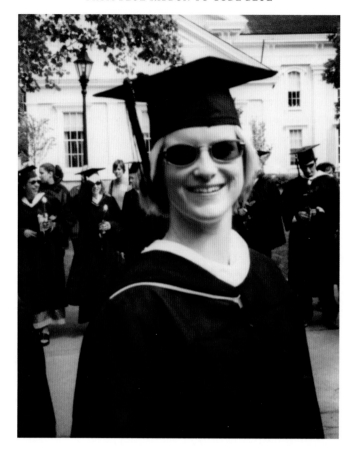

The graduate!

just give me extensions and extra help—Wheaton took a chance on me. I am forever grateful to the college and the community for taking the risk.

In May of 2000, the president of Wheaton College handed me my diploma with the words *magna cum laude* written at the top. Family and friends surrounded me on graduation day. I had really done it. The journey was difficult to the end, but through hard work, determination, and with only a few bumps along the way (like the thumb incident!), I found my way. I also had the most beautiful opportunity in the world: on my graduation day, I looked out on the audience and saw my grandmother, who was battling cancer at the time, beaming with pride during the ceremony.

Evelyn Staudinger

I first met Jen right after she arrived at Wheaton. I had learned that a student who had suffered a traumatic brain injury was coming to campus, and I wanted to get to know her right away because a very dear friend of mine had suffered a TBI a few years earlier, and I had been very much involved in his recovery. From the very beginning, I felt that I could empathize with her and with her need to create a new life for herself.

Our first meeting created an instant bond. Here was a young woman who had just learned to navigate a totally new world and now she was attempting college. To me, she already seemed to have it all together. Jen was one of the most mature young women that I taught at Wheaton. I got to know her very well during her four years there; by the time she graduated, I had come to think that if I had ever had a daughter, I would have wanted her to be like Jen. She was just that special—to me, and to other people as well.

One of the first things that I noticed about Jen was the joy with which she approached everything in life. I thought that was extraordinary with everything she had gone through. The second thing was her determination to excel in all of her courses without wanting or needing any sort of extra help. The third thing that always comes to mind is the dignity with which she carried herself. I had learned that people with traumatic brain injuries are called "the walking wounded." You can't always see or understand how hard they have to work to learn or to navigate the world. The signs of Jen's past trauma were visible, yet once you met her you never noticed them, probably because Jen was completely unselfconscious. Her immediate desire was to make other people feel comfortable.

I didn't treat Jen differently from other students; she didn't want to be treated differently. Art history was a discipline that she adored and had an affinity for; she was incredibly creative. I think creativity helps in the healing process because it takes you out of yourself and away from worries; it helps you focus on the present and helps you understand the great potential you have inside. Jen progressed beautifully because she used the same traits she called upon in her recovery to become a wonderful student. She was determined to get her degree. She was determined to get to graduation day.

Jen lives beautifully in the present. When things in my life are difficult, I always think about how she has created a new world for herself—with emphasis on the word *created*. And she has not only made herself a better person, but others become better for having known her.

Chapter 12

My Gramma: Force of Nature

WHILE MUCH OF THE STRENGTH AND DETERMINATION I called upon during my recovery can probably be attributed to my years of training and competing on horses, I don't think that explains it all. My mother shares those same traits, as she showed in all her efforts to uncover new therapies to help me, and in her resolve to take me to wherever I needed to be. And behind both of us, there was my grandmother.

Gramma was a force of nature, for me and for many others. She and I had an incredible bond. There was a spiritual connection between us that was so very special that it can barely be described in words. Joanne Bass Field Bross was a spellbinding and charming woman who always influenced the lives of those people who came into contact with her. She was not only my grandmother, the woman I loved to be with, but she also had a tremendous impact on my life. She was the one I turned to at different times in my life when I needed her sage advice, which was always so sensible and always seemed to provide just the right answer to my problem. She was the person I wanted to be most like. She was my rock.

A few months after my graduation, my mom and I went to visit Gramma, who we feared was at the end of her battle with non-Hodgkin lymphoma. After spending a few days with her in Virginia, I left to return to Boston to see my boyfriend. I had just boarded the plane when something made me freeze in the aisle. The heavy door of American Flight 593 was about to close when I stepped away from my seat, grabbed my bag, and ran to the front of the plane exclaiming, "I have to get off this plane right now!"

In a very calm and controlled voice, the flight attendant said, "Please return to your seat and fasten your seat belt."

"You don't understand," I told her. "My grandmother is very ill, and I need to be with her! I have to get off this plane."

Everyone else was pushing past me and making their way to their seats, but only one thought kept going through my mind: "What if Gramma passes away and you are not there? You would never forgive yourself." Now, this was a very weird thing to

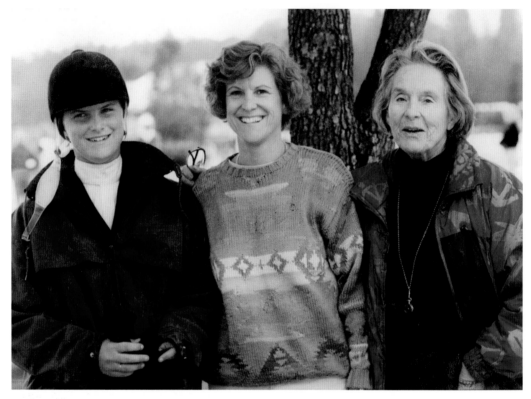

Three generations: Jennifer, Joanne, and Gramma

be saying to myself, considering that just that morning she had seemed to be doing better, and we'd been making plans for the following summer! For some reason, though, I felt a sudden foreboding—as if she were calling to me. Something in me simply knew I had to get off that plane. Finally, the reluctant attendants opened the door and let me make my way up the jetway.

After my taxi arrived back at Gramma's house, I went straight in the back door and through the kitchen. My mom and our friend Sue just stared at me, wondering if they were seeing things. They may have said something to me, but I didn't hear them. I just walked with a purpose, up the kelly green-carpeted staircase (*so* like Gramma's taste), and down the long, narrow hallway to her bedroom.

I had thought it would be okay to leave. My mom, Uncle Peter, Cousin Posy, and our two friends Sue and Brenda had all been at Gramma's house for days. Sue, Posy, and Brenda had flown down from Peterborough just for the day, but it seemed like they too felt an unspoken sense of urgency and didn't leave. Although Gramma claimed she didn't want people around, I think she enjoyed the action. Other people seemed to have a sense of what was happening as well. Every few hours, the doorbell would ring with another flower delivery.

"Hi, Gramma!" I said, entering her bedroom.

"Didn't you leave for Boston?" she asked.

"Oh, my flight was canceled," I said nonchalantly. I couldn't quite describe the true reason I had returned, because I didn't even understand it myself. I only knew that I had this desperate need to be with her at that moment.

I lay down on her bed, and together we listened to Dick Francis's *Longshot* on tape. The words seemed to travel through my brain without sticking—just floating, empty words. All I really cared about was being with my grandmother, who was such an incredible inspiration to me. Lying next to her gave me an overwhelming sense of peace. I knew that this was where I was supposed to be.

I spent as much time as I could with Gramma, talking and listening to books on tape with her, patting her dogs, and trying to get her to eat a little bit. We celebrated her eighty-fifth birthday on Wednesday, July 12. She insisted we go into town and buy caviar and champagne. Gramma and I had a very special tradition that we'd been observing since I was three—we would always bake my mother's birthday cake together. Mom told me that my grandmother used to say that she had never seen a child with my kind of concentration and patience. So now, on my gramma's birthday in McLean, Virginia, I made a birthday cake alone, with the best chocolate frosting ever! Even though she wasn't eating much, I thought if I baked a wonderful, delicious, chocolate birthday cake, she might take a few bites. Gramma loved it.

The evening of July 13, she told her son Peter, a doctor, that she was in a lot of pain. He had promised her she wouldn't have to suffer, and he upped her morphine drip. Later, she fell into a comatose state of heavy breathing. Gramma had begun to slip away. The next night, we all surrounded her bed. Together as a family, we told her, "Go peacefully, it is okay. You are loved and will always be loved." I was holding her hand as she took her last breath in the middle of the night.

I walked back to my room and cried myself to sleep. The next morning, when no one was around, I went back to her room to say goodbye. I told her how much I loved her and that she would forever be a part of my life. "You are an amazing woman, Gramma, and you will always be my inspiration. Thank you for calling me back from the plane. I was so glad to be here with you. I love you."

Gramma

What an amazing life Joanne Bass Field Bross led! Born in 1912 in Peterborough, New Hampshire, she became an artist, studying sculpture and painting in Paris, and she maintained a very active social life. While in Paris, she met the famous art dealer Amboise Vollard, who spent time showing her art. She especially liked Renoir. She remembered being taken into a basement where hundreds of paintings by artists such as Cezanne, Renoir, and Manet were stacked against the wall, waiting for someone to buy them.

By all accounts, she was exceptional, beautiful, outspoken, and charismatic, with a devil-may-care attitude. She was not haughty, but she acted as if rules and laws didn't apply to her. She played the part of a naughty girl, and always liked getting away with something. She had a strong belief in her opinions. She often felt others didn't know what they were doing—and she told them so. In addition to a strong personality, Joanne remembers her mother had a reputation for her sixth sense; some even whispered she was a witch.

Ever the world traveler, she visited Egypt while in her twenties and spent time with an Egyptologist who was doing research for *National Geographic.* She worked hard but she also had fun. She told stories of riding horseback on the sand in the moonlight around the Pyramids. She lived for a time in New York City, at the Mews on lower Fifth Avenue near Washington Square Park, where she continued to study art. She moved in interesting circles—while she was visiting Hearst Castle in San Simeon, California, a face appeared in the window of her room. It was Charlie Chaplin, and she spent the rest of the evening with him.

She met Marshall Field while visiting Harvard with a friend. From Chicago, he was one of the most eligible bachelors in the country and she went on to marry him—but not before mesmerizing suitors in Peterborough. She said she intended to have "their eyes spinning in their heads." Joanne remembers a story told to her when she was a teenager by an older man at a party, who said, "You're Joanne Bass's daughter? Your mother was the most beautiful woman I ever saw!" He recounted a rapturous story about her mother out fishing with a few beaus, wearing a dress with buttons all down its front. And she said to the beaus, "For every fish you catch, you can bite a button off my dress!" When Joanne later

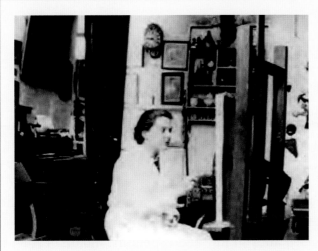

Gramma in her Paris studio

asked her mother if the story was true, her mother said, "Yes! It was great fun." (She also told teenaged Joanne that if she didn't have at least five or six boyfriends at a time, she "wasn't doing it right.") After marrying Marshall Field, Joanne moved to Charlottesville, Virginia, where Marshall attended law school at the University of Virginia. They spent many nights dining with Franklin Delano Roosevelt, whose son was a classmate.

For all her sophistication Joanne was a country girl at heart—she loved animals and she liked keeping chickens and ducks wherever she lived. Family lore has it that one warm day while living on Long Island, she was painting her upstairs bathroom naked when she heard a terrible racket outside. She looked out the window to see that all of her ducks had marched over from the barn and were going wild. She threw some clothes on and ran outside to see what the matter was, only to find that the house was on fire. She liked to think the ducks saved her life.

She's remembered for riding fast with her hair streaming out behind her. She had very little fear and lots of ability. She could ride to the hunt sidesaddle; she showed horses and rode trails. A fabulous tennis player and a beautiful horsewoman, her name appears on several tennis trophies at the Dublin Lake Club in New Hampshire. Supposedly, when she had lost the first set of a tennis tournament 6–0, and was down 5–2 in the second set, her second husband, John Bross, left the event assuming she would lose and be home soon. He mixed up a batch of martinis to lift her spirits and then waited . . . and waited . . . and waited. Finally, she burst through the door and, to his amazement, announced that she had fought her way back to win the match!

Chapter 13

CALIFORNIA (HERE I COME)

Indulge every creative whim—
It is incredibly healing.
from *A Distant Memory*

DURING MY SENIOR YEAR AT WHEATON, I began dating a man named Rohit, who lived in Cambridge, Massachusetts. After I graduated, my plan was to stay in Boston to be with him. My Gramma passed away in July and I spent the month of August searching for a rental apartment in Boston. My real estate broker, Joe, kept talking about "pulling the triggah"—signing a contract. I finally did "pull the triggah" and rented an apartment on Beacon Street.

Moving in, my mom helped me outfit the apartment with furniture and knick-knacks from Crate and Barrel. The apartment was cute and comfortable, and I was happy to call it home. I was expecting Rohit to move in too, but when he arrived, he was distant and noncommittal. When he saw that I had unpacked some of his things and hung his clothes in the closet with mine, he unexpectedly panicked. That was the beginning of the end. It soon became clear that Rohit didn't want to be there, and I was left alone.

The main problem when he left was that I didn't know what to do with myself. I didn't have a job, and I didn't know of any job that I could get. I had no sense of direction, and I ended up constantly walking up and down Newbury Street in search of the best lattes and scones in Boston. I was lonely, and I took in roommates in an attempt to fill the void. None of them worked out. There was a high-end cooking store several blocks from my apartment, and I walked there almost every day to visit the manager, Scotty, who somehow, sadly, became my only friend. I also tried my hand at cooking school—anything to fit in and feel normal, but I ended up cutting my finger badly because of my tremor. Still, I decided I wanted to become a pastry chef.

My uncle owned a company based in Boston, and one of his employees, Juan Prieto, invited me to a cocktail party one evening. I accepted gladly. Among the guests there, I met Nathalie Graber, a yoga teacher who taught a method called Forrest Yoga.

I began taking classes with Nathalie and studied with her for a few months, which was very therapeutic for me in many ways. I became fascinated by this extremely challenging form of yoga. At the end of one class, Nathalie pulled me aside and said, "There's a yoga teacher training course in Santa Monica taught by Ana Forrest, the developer of Forrest Yoga. I think you would really benefit from taking it."

I remember wandering up Newbury Street, weighing my options. Should I go to Burgundy, France, and become a pastry chef? Or should I go to California and study yoga? Ultimately, California won, mostly because I was on a mission to better myself, to become fully healed, and I knew yoga would do that for me—not so much pastries! I was delighted when Ana Forrest accepted me into her teacher training class despite my brain injury. I packed my things, said goodbye to the East Coast, and made the long journey to California alone.

Ana Forrest, an internationally recognized pioneer in yoga and emotional healing, has been changing people's lives for nearly forty years. Ana created Forrest Yoga while working through healing from her own life trauma. Forrest Yoga is an intensely physical, internally focused practice that emphasizes how to carry a transformative experience off the mat and into daily life.

Before enrolling in Ana's course, I first spent a month at the Optimum Health Institute in Lemon Grove, California. That month was filled mostly with a raw diet, wheatgrass, and colonics—I was trying to clean myself out before I immersed myself in the yoga world. Part of the aim of that cleanse was losing weight. My life in Boston had been yoga-oriented, but yoga had been coupled with my never-ending quest to find the best scones and lattes in town. I ended up staying on the raw diet for about a year.

At the end of that month, I returned to Santa Monica to meet my mother, who came to help me move in. I had rented a room from a woman named Brigitte, a member of the Forrest Yoga Studio. Brigitte was French, and she was also on a raw diet. My mom bonded with her even more than I did—maybe because she was hoping that Brigitte would watch over me.

Before my first training session, I introduced myself to Ana Forrest and told her about my situation. Despite my insecurities, she was very excited to work with me. I remember so vividly meeting her for the first time; we formed an immediate connection. Even more exciting was that I was becoming more independent. College had been great for my independence, but it was definitely a transition phase. Now, I was living across the country, away from my mother and my New Hampshire home. It felt amazing.

Forrest Yoga is based on holding a position for an extended amount of time, and it fit my situation better than traditional yoga, which can involve speed and balance. In Forrest Yoga, I could take as much time as I wanted. At the beginning of my time with Ana, I was asked to do Downward Dog, a basic yoga pose. The movement is pretty simple, but I was too weak to hold the position. My biggest accomplishment, by far, was conquering a pose called Wheel. Wheel, a more complicated pose, is similar to a backbend, and for me to even push up from the floor to get into that position seemed impossible. Soon enough, though, I was holding my weight.

After I completed my teacher training, I became an Ana Forrest groupie and followed her around the country. Ana and I developed a close friendship during our travels and work together. She invited me to see the house she was building with her husband Jonathan on Orcas Island, off the coast of northern Washington. I felt so honored that she wanted to share her amazing new house with me. She had just begun construction and I stayed in a camper on the property. We practiced yoga together every morning.

After I helped Jennifer move in with Brigitte, I flew back to New Hampshire. Jennifer would call and talk about her class and the ease of living in Santa Monica. She loved the great climate and it was easier to pursue her raw diet there. During one of these phone calls, I realized she was going to move there permanently.

A month later Jennifer called and said, "Mom, guess what?"

Of course, I knew what. "What?" I asked, humoring her.

"I've decided to move to Santa Monica and find an apartment here."

"I knew you would!" I said.

"How did you know?" Jennifer inquired.

"Because I would move there too, if I were you."

I benefitted hugely from my experience with Forrest Yoga, but over time, I realized that I didn't want to become a yoga teacher. My real mission was to keep moving and discovering the next therapy that would aid me on my journey of recovery. After talking to my mom, we both came to the conclusion that I needed to work more intensely again with Emilie Conrad and Continuum.

I found my own apartment to rent on Ocean Boulevard, with a view of the ocean. I was one block away from my good friends Chantalynn and Clay, whom I'd met the year before. They told my mom that they'd watch out for me. Later, I bought a small apartment four blocks away on Fourth Street. Santa Monica is spread out and it has a great public transportation system, but I couldn't always take the bus, so during those early years I had a number of assistants who drove me places and helped me run errands.

Jason Micallef, personal assistant

I met Jennifer by chance in a coffee shop in Santa Monica. She and her assistant and I got to chatting—I studied art in college, so we had something in common. One thing led to another, and when it became clear that her assistant couldn't keep working for her, Jen offered me the position.

Jen couldn't drive because of her vision difficulties, so I drove her to physical therapy, to get groceries, and I helped out with whatever errands she needed. At the time, I was writing for a living, so it fit me well; I could drop her off, write for a few hours while she did whatever she needed to do, and then drive her to her next appointment or back home. It was a great fit, and I loved the time I got to spend talking with her.

During the two years I worked for Jen, she made astounding leaps in her recovery. I met her relatively far into the process, but even those two years made a huge difference. The first time we met, her speech was slurred and her eyes were unfocused, but those issues improved every day.

I'm impressed with the change in Jen's emotional fortitude. One of the biggest differences I see is her ability to curb her frustrations and work through problems now. Her speech has picked up almost to the point where she can think and talk at the same rate. She's blossomed into a very communicative motivational speaker. It's hard to believe that this woman who reveals her life on a stage in front of hundreds is the same one who suffered a life-changing accident so many years ago.

Once I moved in, I became obsessed with Continuum Movement, practicing eight to ten hours a day. I was singularly focused on Continuum, my health, and watching *Sex and the City*. I ate only vegetables and two-and-a-half ounces of protein per meal each day. I remember lying in my bed in tears, not knowing what to do with myself. Simply put, I was depressed. I didn't feel like my life had any purpose.

I'd taken some studio art classes when I was at Wheaton to fulfill the requirement for the art history major and later I began painting seriously, after attending a workshop in Florida with Graham Nickson, who ran the New York Studio School. When I settled in California I took lessons from Barbra Mindell, a wonderful local artist and a Continuum teacher. Painting became a way for me to express myself. I created a painting of galloping horses, and it symbolized for me the power and strength I needed to overcome my challenges. The painting was constructed from a series of clippings that I had cut out of a magazine. As I was working on it, I came to realize that this painting had a double meaning for me: the loss of my life as an equestrian atop a powerful animal, but also the remembrance of the power and strength Gramma showed during her long and arduous battle with cancer. I began to look at my paintings differently, and with each one I completed, I learned more about my new self.

Art has been a major contributor to my healing process. I've kept up with my poetry, and writing has put me more in touch with my feelings of loss and acceptance. I've been able to work through many of my internal and external problems by expressing myself on paper. Through creative expression I have been better able to reach a certain peace, and to understand and accept the new person I have become.

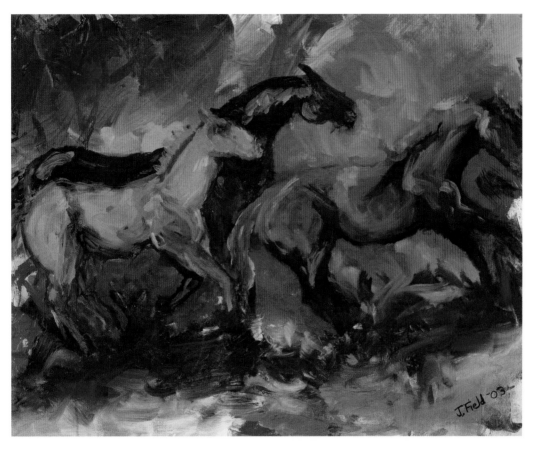

Jennifer's painting, " A Distant Memory"

As I emerged from a two-month-long coma
and was confronted by the extent of my injuries,
I remember thinking it was not worth it to fight—
that there was no way to recover.
And the doctors agreed.
But my mother had a different plan—as mothers often do!
She said, "You will regain control of your body,
and you will move forward in your life by finding a new path."
Sometimes when you face a wall,
you have to turn your focus in a new direction.
There's always another way
and you have to try as many things as possible
in order to find the path that's right for you.

from *A Distant Memory*

Chapter 14

CREATING *A DISTANT MEMORY*

WHEN A FRIEND SUGGESTED I APPLY to the Ruskin School of Acting in Santa Monica, I looked at him like he was crazy. "Acting?" I said, bewildered. "*Me?* I know this is California, but that is not what I came here for."

He persisted, and eventually I took his suggestion into serious consideration. He told me that even if I didn't want to become an actress, this particular program, which used the Meisner Technique, might help me tremendously.

He was right. After interviewing with John Ruskin, I knew that although the program might be difficult, it would ultimately be very rewarding. Sanford Meisner, creator of the Meisner Technique, says that acting is "living truthfully under imaginary circumstances," and his technique was founded on that philosophy. "I can do that," I thought. "Maybe."

Meisner believed that what happens on stage is all about the other person. If you listen and react to your partner's behavior, rather than focusing on your own internal thoughts and feelings, you get authentic behavior.

To my delight, I was fortunate enough to be accepted to the Ruskin School. There, I completed a three-year training course in the Meisner Technique. Acting class allowed me, with all of my challenges, to just be myself and talk. There were various stages of the work, one of which was working with an impediment. I was assigned Tourette syndrome and autism, and I found out very quickly that I was able to embody someone with a neurological disability very well. Everyone in the class struggled with this section, but it proved to be my favorite because, again, I was just me!

Another assignment was based on a book of poetry called *Spoon River Anthology*. Various sections of the poem were given to each student to interpret on their own. I believed the lines I had been given should be acted out like a caterpillar emerging from a cocoon and morphing into a butterfly, which symbolically told my story. I felt this showed my journey from feeling ugly and entrapped, to being free and able to soar. The Meisner Technique allowed my acting to be about me—my life and my history.

The Meisner Technique also included memorizing a script by eliminating all punctuation and just saying the words aloud in one complete sentence. This method proved to be very helpful for me, largely because it took "thinking" out of the memorization and performance, and made it into something automatic. I learned to take less time speaking, and to stop slurring my words and enunciate. The best part of this particular form of "therapy" was that it wasn't the same kind of tedium as putting clothespins on a ruler; I loved what I was doing, and I was passionate about the message I could convey.

Meisner's technique also involved verbal repetition and noticing expressions. The verbal repetition was based on speed, which proved to be a challenge for a girl who'd lost a lot of her ability to speak only a few years before. A part of my brain had been taken away from me, and this new technique provided a way for me to get it back. As time went on, I gained confidence, and the program ended up being a wonderful help in my recovery. For my final scene at the end of my last year I played Laura from *The Glass Menagerie* by Tennessee Williams, a very shy girl with an emotional disorder. I loved playing this part and received many compliments. I was thrilled when John Ruskin personally congratulated me. My friend Sue, who watched my performance later on DVD said, "Don't take this the wrong way, but I was really surprised you were so good."

I remember flying out for Jennifer's final performance. I couldn't believe that I was going to be attending a scene with my daughter portraying Laura from **The Glass Menagerie**! *My mind kept going back to that girl who had fought so hard after her accident to take her first steps, to this girl standing proudly on the stage in front of me. It was hard to believe. She was building a life for herself and I couldn't have been more thrilled!*

During my time at the Ruskin School, I went to see a one-man show by Paul Linke called *Time Flies When You're Alive*. At the end of the show, I came out of the audience and said to John Ruskin, "That is what I want to do! I want to develop my own one-woman show."

"Yeah, sure, Jen, that would be great," he said, not really believing I was serious, or that I could possibly do it. Actually, I didn't quite believe that I was serious either, but that familiar feeling of determination came over me.

I called my mom and told her that I had finally found the thing that I wanted to

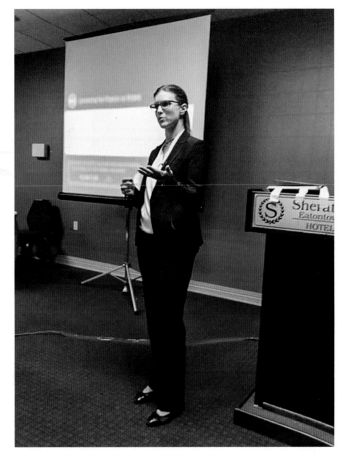

Delivering the keynote speech in front of a corporate audience

do. She was enthusiastic as always, but I wasn't convinced that she thought it would happen. I *knew* it would.

During my final year of acting school, a teacher of mine, Michael Laurie, suggested we work together on my own one-woman show about my accident and my recovery. I'd been writing for years to sort out my feelings, and now someone was actually saying to me that everything I'd experienced on my journey could be said aloud and used to help others. I wondered if my story could actually inspire and help other people.

I remember going to Michael's apartment one day with stacks and stacks of my medical records and poetry, and just dumping everything on the floor.

Michael Laurie, Meisner Technique instructor

I became Jen's temporary driver in 2004 while her usual helper (a friend of mine) was out of town for a couple of weeks. All I was told was that Jennifer was recovering from a brain injury, would need help running errands, and was very sweet and easy to work with.

After a few errands and a visit to an acupuncturist, we got onto the subject of writing and Jen read me some poems that she had written. It occurred to me that they might be gathered into a book, but after hearing the whole story of Jen's accident and recovery, it was obvious that she should write a one-woman show that she could perform. Although the idea excited her, the thought of performing seemed ridiculous to her. At the time, Jen's speech and physical movements were still slow and deliberate. But she agreed to try, so we started writing, she joined an acting class, and *A Distant Memory* was born.

Throughout the years of writing and developing the show, and after seeing the performance that followed, I got to witness Jen's courage and commitment. She faced many challenges and took them all in stride. I watched her develop physically, verbally, emotionally, and professionally as an actress during that time. It truly changed her life and continues to change the lives of those that experience it. My involvement certainly changed mine.

"I can't deal with all of this anymore!" I said, overwhelmed. "Please. Help me."

He spent days trying to sort through everything. We even interviewed the people who were closest to me in the hospital and during my rehabilitation. After a full year of working together almost every day, we had developed my one-woman show, *A Distant Memory*. My knowledge of the Meisner Technique allowed me to put together something intimate, honest, and important.

The first time I performed *A Distant Memory* was in 2005 at the Ruskin Group Theatre in Santa Monica. The performance was raw and unpolished. I performed the show sitting down, and when I'd get up to demonstrate something, I would often nearly fall over. I still didn't have a great memory, and back then it took me months of daily practice to memorize the script. During the show, I would often lose my place and need a lot of prompting. It was a rough start, but I got a standing ovation.

When I walked off stage at the end of the show, the first person I saw was John Ruskin, the director of the theatre, and I said to him, "I have found it! The feeling I had while on a horse entering the ring, all eyes upon me. I never thought I would have that feeling of excitement and anticipation again without being on a horse." It was a glorious moment to realize that thrill was still attainable for me.

After that first performance, my neighbor wrote me a note, telling me how courageous she thought I was to perform in front of all those people. I didn't necessarily feel brave; I was just back in the ring again.

Jennifer was scheduled to perform her show four times at the Ruskin Group Theatre. For some reason she didn't want me to come until the third show. There she was in the middle of the stage with the audience all around her. She started speaking, the audience was rapt, and my mind traveled back to a moment in the hospital when she was still in a coma. I was watching her intently, trying to see inside of her, and in that second, I composed a poem of my own for her, a mantra really for us both to hold on to. It goes like this:

I can catch any leaf
And I can touch any cloud
And if I cannot do it today
I will do it tomorrow

And there she was center stage, touching the clouds. She had done it.

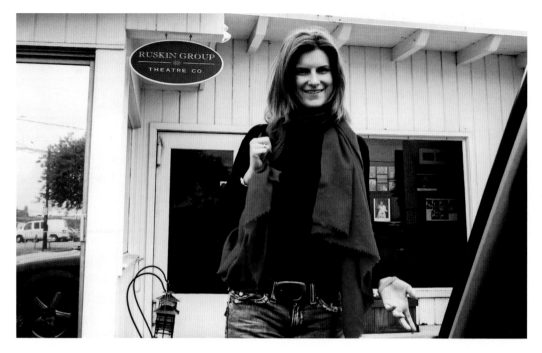

In front of the Ruskin Group Theatre Company

The creation of my one-woman show was the beginning of my speaking career. I knew in that moment that I wanted to bring my speech to many audiences around the country, and to people with head injuries in particular. I hoped my story could inspire them to overcome their obstacles and never give up. I wanted to give back, and to that end I created the J. Field Foundation and received my 501(c)(3) status.

Performing *A Distant Memory* has also been a continuous source of therapy for me. My voice has been pushed beyond limits it could never have reached with just speech therapy. With each show that I deliver, I feel that a little piece of my trauma drops away.

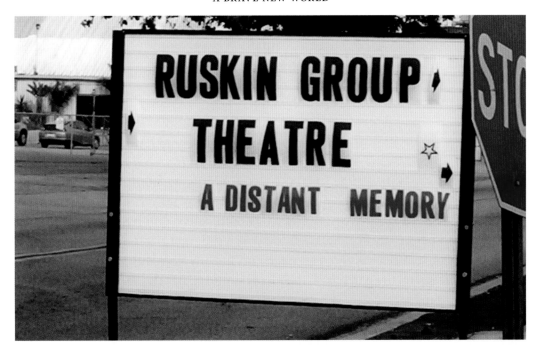

John Ruskin, founder of the Ruskin School of Acting

After she saw *Time Flies When You're Alive*, I could tell Jennifer was enthusiastic about the concept of a one-woman show. She worked with one of the teachers at our school, and we ran *A Distant Memory* for the first time while she was doing her two-year program on the Meisner Technique. We loved her, we loved her story, and we loved the inspirational spirit that she brought to the stage, the school, and the other students.

To put together a one-woman show is difficult for anyone, but to create this show with Jen's challenges is evidence of the spirit of her message: it is possible to overcome unbeatable obstacles. Many people go through struggles and end up defeated, but she used her struggles as motivation. Jennifer is an inspiration, both as an artist and as a human being.

Chapter 15

The New Normal

Choose to try more than you quit.
You will succeed more than you fail.
from *A Distant Memory*

MY PERCEPTION OF THE WORLD TODAY is completely different from the way I experienced it before my accident; Jen today is a different person from Jen pre-accident. I was once a self-centered teenage girl, but my accident humbled me. As I walk down the street, my gait has changed, my thinking has changed, and what I see, literally, has changed.

I don't think of these changes as negative. They created opportunities and put me on the path that I am meant to be on.

The night before Jennifer's accident, I was up late, packing for the next day's trip to New York. After I finished packing, I went upstairs to say goodnight to her, and I saw as I approached her bedroom door that the light was still on. When I opened the door, I saw that she was on the telephone.

"It's eleven o'clock at night, and you're on the phone?" I said. "Have you done your homework yet?"

"No, I haven't," she said, covering the receiver.

"Well, you need to get off the phone and do your homework, then," I responded, slightly irritated.

Jennifer, such a typical teenage girl at the time, snapped back, "You can't make me, and I'm going to talk on the phone as long as I want."

I walked right up to her, looked her in the eye, and stated, "I am your mother, I can make you do it—and don't you forget it."

As Jen glared at me, a little voice in my head warned me that this could be one of those battles I might not win, so I left her there. The next day, though, Jennifer called me from school. She had talked to her trainer and they couldn't get the horses down to the riding ring because of the freezing rain. She told me she was *going to spend a little more time at school and then come home.*

"Have a wonderful time in New York, Mom," she said before we hung up. "I'm going to miss you, and I love you."

"I love you too," I said carefully. "Wait a minute," I thought as I hung up the phone. "What's this all about?"

I can't even remember the girl my mother is talking about. I've changed. I had no choice but to embrace that life does indeed change.

It took me years to understand my accident was actually a positive force in my life. My mother and I have the same conversation over and over again where I tell her how fortunate I feel that I endured such an injury, even though I wouldn't wish it on anyone else. She always asks, "How can you feel lucky after such a devastating accident?" My mother's perspective on my accident and recovery is different from mine. While she was on the outside, frantically trying to get me well, I was, at first, on a little cotton cloud inside, just doing what I was told.

As I got better, I began to see that I just might achieve my goal. At first it was to get well, get back on a horse, and get back to who I was. But slowly I realized and accepted that could never happen. I couldn't return to who I was before the accident. I had to accept my injury before I could become the person I wanted to be. I understood that I was not a victim. I did not want to feel sorry for myself.

Then the goal became trying to figure out who the new me was. I have been shaped by this life-altering trauma and the journey towards recovery. Inch by inch by inch, I am finding the things that define the new me. But most of all, I want to share my message of hope and inspiration to help others as they face unbearable obstacles.

It was a saving grace for me that in the early years of my therapies, I never really noticed how people saw me. I just marched forward, my eyes on the prize. My friend Sue reminds me about the time she took me to the bookstore at Keene State College to get books for my writing class. We laughed and talked the whole way over, because she was used to the way in which I spoke softly, haltingly, and even drifting off during a conversation. Once we got to the bookstore, the clerk kept addressing Sue as if I were incapable of talking, which annoyed Sue who kept saying to him, "Ask *her*. Ask Jen."

As Sue tells me, she'd spent enough time with me to know that if somebody just slowed down and listened to me, it was clear that I was very much there, even if

Joanne Matz, golf instructor

About five years ago Jennifer came down to Jupiter Island and took her first golf lesson. I was fascinated by what had happened to her and amazed that she was even thinking about hitting a golf ball. She had very poor balance at that time, and I was afraid she was going to fall down. She'd take a swing and almost fall backward because she couldn't hold the finish.

Jennifer never looked at golf as something she wasn't able to do. The first year, I was really set on trying to get her to be able to see the ball, because of her double vision. I never treated her any differently as a student; I had to find out exactly what I needed to know to make her able to swing. I would ask, "Where do you see the ball, here or there? Which side?"

Jen worked at golf every year, and every year she got so much better. I think the practice helped her. I also think the positive experience of doing something that should have been almost impossible gave her a little more confidence. When she walks up to the tee today, you would not know anything had ever happened to her. Five years ago, you would have thought, "Oh, my god! *She's* going to hit a golf ball?" I told her about the first day when I was afraid she was going to fall down—and she laughed. She's such a good sport. I think that's one of the reasons why she's done so well.

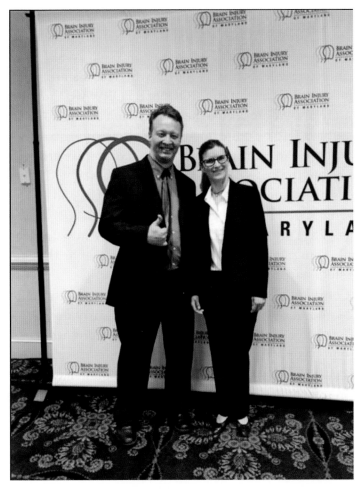

Speaking to the Brain Injury Association in Maryland

exterior gestures and slowness of speech indicated that I might not be. The clerk's perception of me, though, was that I couldn't answer even the most basic of questions. I was completely unaware of how he saw me, and felt I was communicating effectively with him.

I'm grateful that I missed his reaction to me. One of the keys to my recovery has been being oblivious to how people perceive me. Ironically, this has enabled me to move forward much less self-consciously. Even today, many things go over my head, but maybe that's a good thing.

As time goes on, I continually ask myself, what is "normal?" Everyone has his or her own idea of "normal." I had thought I wanted to get back to the person I had been.

My friend and colleague, Sam Cawthorn, who lost his arm in an automobile accident, has trademarked the phrase "BOUNCE FORWARD," and thinking about it has helped me greatly. We are used to hearing "bounce *back*" to refer to our return to normalcy. Sam says, "To be quite honest, this phrase is . . . completely wrong, as it implies that we have had a struggle or a crisis, and now we are bouncing back to where we were before the crisis. This is . . . reactive thinking." He believes that we should stop focusing on and talking about bouncing back, and instead bounce *forward* into a new life, a new beginning—a new normal.

In some ways, I feel my body and mind have actually surpassed who I once was. At the same time, I am saddened to know that I will never be the competitor that I was on a horse. But I have found a new way to compete.

I now think of every obstacle that I encounter as a competition to win. On the day that I walked into Michael Laurie's apartment with all of my poetry and writing, there was a driving force behind me to work on my one-woman show. I knew that I could inspire people through my story to pursue their own recovery. I was "bouncing forward." Sometimes, I imagined myself bouncing on my large physioball, bouncing from one new experience to the next and finally into my new life. It made me smile. The only way I could thrive in this new world was to create a new normal for myself—to be a new person in a new world.

In the early stages of my recovery, my mother consulted a psychic in California. Among other things, he told my mom that I would live, and that I would get better because I was here for a purpose. He said that in my future I would teach and inspire people.

At the time, it gave my mother hope and reassurance. I've thought about that a lot over the past several years. I was given another chance at life. I don't think my accident was just bad luck; I honestly believe it was meant to be. When someone has an accident and they lose so much, often they say, "I wish I could just go back in time and do all those things I never got to do." I don't feel that. I don't feel that at all.

It's not that I'm *glad* that I was in an accident that November, but I'm not unhappy. It helped, certainly, that the universe had let me have a successful end to my riding career. But what happened, happened; it turned out to be a gift in a lot of ways. It's given me far more meaning in my life. I have the drive to do something greater, to touch others.

To that end, my one-woman show has evolved into my work as a motivational speaker. I have delivered my speech at many Brain Injury Alliance events, graduations, schools, and colleges, and in corporate settings. These experiences have been as thrilling as riding in the ring. But this time, I'm giving back.

There have been times when I've forgotten a line or fallen silent for a few seconds, not knowing where to go. My brain doesn't work like other people's brains. I'm unable to ad lib if I forget a line; I just see a blank wall. If I wait too long, though, it starts to make the audience nervous. Today, the words usually come back in time; in case they don't, I try to have a prompter nearby to cue me.

When I'm speaking, whether I'm stuck or flowing effortlessly, my goal is not for my audience to feel bad for me. I don't want or need sympathy. I want my listeners to empathize, to be able to learn from my experience, and to never give up on their goals. Simply put: if I can do it, you can do it too.

Lou Heckler, motivational speaker and coach

I have had the good fortune of knowing and working with Jennifer for a number of years. She is a person of great heart, fine intelligence, and tremendous perseverance. By making the progress that she has, she's beautifully demonstrated why one should never take "no" for an answer, especially when it comes to one's own well being.

No one should have to go through the years of treatments and hard work that she had to endure since her horrific accident, but she managed to do it with the grace and strength that she applies to everything else in her life. She came to me for help in smoothing out the bumps in a lecture about her life-changing experience. I was impressed to see her keen interest in making improvements on what was already a very good presentation. This is the trait of a true champion, and I believe it was ingrained in her from her earliest days in her equestrian competitions. I've also had the privilege of meeting Jen's mother, who has worked tirelessly and purposefully on behalf of her daughter. Throughout Jennifer's journey, Joanne accompanied her to countless programs, clinics, and adventures, always sure that she could help make her daughter whole again.

I believe in the power of love. I believe in the indomitable human spirit. I believe we all need to play the hand we're dealt. I've met no one else who exemplifies these beliefs better than Jennifer Field.

Chapter 16

FULL CIRCLE

I REMEMBER SO CLEARLY SITTING IN A CAFÉ, thinking I wanted to write about my journey to recovery. I wanted to talk about the amazing therapists and alternative energy healers that I've worked with. Looking back, I realize my hope was that others who found themselves in a similar situation could benefit from my experience. My keynote speech is designed to give guidance and inspiration. The J. Field Foundation was created with the goal of providing funding, hope, and healing to those with brain injuries. All I can wish for is that my story inspires people to never give up or give in.

As you know now from having read these pages, my recovery was not instantaneous or a miracle. It was never easy. I've worked and struggled on my journey, inch by inch by inch, and the end result is that I'm standing, speaking, and just maybe changing one small part of the world, one person at a time. As counterintuitive as it might sound, I'm really very grateful for every challenge that has been laid out before me. I can't believe that it's been over twenty years since I awoke from a coma and found myself in a blue padded room, unable to walk, talk, or move my right arm. I want my victory to be known and understood by those who find themselves in a similar situation. I want them to know that with hard work, perseverance, and patience, they can succeed as I did.

But what does success really mean? It's not just found in a riding ring or a stadium or even in the writing of a book. It encompasses all aspects of life and love. In a sense, I missed out on many of the early experiences of being a teenager. But luckily for me, that part of my life came full circle when I reconnected with my high school sweetheart, David.

I was a naïve freshman in boarding school when I first met David, a junior who had just arrived from New Jersey. I was fifteen, and easily overcome by the flirtations of an extremely good-looking young man. As a new student and a freshman, I was very unsure of myself but he was so confident.

It was the perfect high school romance. We started dating and holding hands walking to class. He was so sweet; I never felt like he was taking advantage of me or being insincere. On a school trip to New York City together, we snuck off to his father's apartment with two other couples in tow. The other couples lost their virginity, but we just kissed and fooled around and laughed and talked all night. Sadly, because I was riding so much and unable to attend his soccer or lacrosse games David eventually broke off with me. Even though I was upset, I couldn't blame him.

Taylor Swift writes songs about her adventures, misadventures, and past loves. Even though she wrote most of her songs as a teenager, the intensity of the emotion encompasses a whole lifetime. As I think about David now, I can't help but think of her song *Fifteen*: "It's your freshman year, and when you're fifteen and somebody tells you they love you, you're gonna believe them. And when you're fifteen, feeling like there's nothing to figure out, well, count to ten, take it in. This is life before you know who you're gonna be."

David, who I'd been out of touch with for decades, reached out to me through Facebook just to reconnect. As we talked, it became clear he also needed help and guidance.

In the summer of 2011, he had been diagnosed with multiple sclerosis. My heart went out to David as he told me his story, because I understood where he was. I had been through the same questions and looks of uncertainty from everyone near me. I was touched and felt grateful that he was able to reach out, and pleased that I could offer some comfort and guidance. After our initial connection on Facebook and many long emails, we began talking for hours on the phone, almost every day. We were both only looking for a simple laugh to brighten our days, and we found that in each other. As so often is the case when you reconnect with someone from your past, the intervening years just melted away and somehow we were once again teenagers. My mom, overhearing us once, said we sounded like two kids in a sandbox delighting in one another. And it really did have that kind of innocence for a long time.

Through the lessons I have learned from my own recovery, I have found a deep satisfaction in providing comfort and hope to others. In the process of cultivating my career as a public speaker, I frequently meet complete strangers who share stories of their own challenges, and it touches me deeply. I am forever bonded to these strangers through our mutual traumas and recoveries. David is the first person I've known intimately who now faces many of the challenges I've faced.

Many people have told me about their experiences of pain, suffering, courage, and recovery. I never cease to be moved. But nothing brings home the reality of these challenges like the stories of someone you know and care about. My mission in life is to help others overcome seemingly impossible obstacles. Reconnecting with David renewed my commitment to this mission in a very personal way. I felt an immediate connection with my long-lost friend, and I loved being able to help him. No one had really understood what he was going through, and he found in me someone he could talk to about it. Just talking was in itself an amazing therapy for both of us.

One morning in the summer of 2012, I was doing my exercises and replaying a conversation we'd had in my head. I suddenly rose, realizing he and I were planning to be in New York at the same time. I texted him immediately, and the planning began.

I remember being so excited. I hadn't seen David in twenty years, and now we were going to meet for the first time! I was nervous, though—since I hadn't seen him since before my accident, I had no idea what he was going to think of me. I grew more and more nervous, and excited, as the day drew closer.

While I was in New York that weekend, I stayed with my friend Sue in her apartment. The day of our date, I could feel the butterflies in my stomach just fighting to get out. When David rang the buzzer, I stepped up to the door. I could see his face on Sue's video monitor, and I just said, "*Wow*." He was everything I thought he would be, and more. Sue had explained to me how to buzz him into the apartment building, but now I couldn't remember it. I frantically pushed every button I could find, but nothing worked. I could see his face and we were talking on our cell phones, but I couldn't buzz him in. I just couldn't figure it out! Finally, I called for the elevator. Sue had warned me it was the slowest elevator in New York, and the nine floors truly seemed like ninety.

As I approached the lobby, the butterflies in my stomach became even more active. Then the elevator door opened and there was David behind the glass lobby doors, holding up his phone to take my picture. I opened the door, stepped into his arms, and the past twenty years disappeared. We were back in that beautiful high school romance again. As he held me tightly in his arms, he whispered to me, "I will never let you go again."

From there, our relationship grew more intimate. We began to date and our relationship grew stronger. He made me laugh in a way I'd never laughed before. In

2013 when David's divorce became final, I thought for sure he would run into my arms and we would be together forever. The reality was that he was freaked out by the failure of his marriage, his three kids were extremely unhappy and struggling with the situation, and his MS was ever present. Instead of turning to me, he turned inside himself. I realized as the year wore on that we were not going to make it, and I was devastated. When I had reunited with David in New York two years earlier, he had told me, "I'll never let you go again." Yet here he was letting me go. The reconnection was over. The fairytale was over. And I thought I would never meet anyone as perfect as I had believed David was for me.

Chapter 17

Endless Possibilities

TODAY, MY RECOVERY IS STILL ONGOING. To be a successful musician, you have to practice every day. In a way, the body is like an instrument that needs to be tuned. Most recently, we learned about a therapy called Brain State Technology.

Early in 2011, a friend called from Florida to tell me that she'd tried a new therapy and thought Jen would benefit greatly from it. Lee Gerdes of Scottsdale, Arizona, developed software using the brainwaves of two transcendental monks who he believed to have the most balanced brains in the world. He computerized the brainwaves and made the software into the foundation of his treatment, Brain State Technology. I jumped at the opportunity for Jen.

We were fortunate enough to find Shannon Krause, in nearby Bow, New Hampshire, who was trained in Brain State Technology. Although Shannon looked about twenty years old (which kind of freaked me out), she turned out to be extremely skilled. Shannon assessed Jennifer, and then we embarked on ten days of treatment. The normal treatment is two sessions a day for five days, but we decided slower and longer worked better for Jennifer. It involves attaching electrodes to different areas of your head to track your brain waves while you read, open and close your eyes, partially focus your eyes, and do other things. Computer software translates the brain waves into sound that is played back to you through headphones, making you very calm and relaxed. During the process, your brain becomes rebalanced; when the brain is balanced, the result is, as Lee Gerdes says, "'A Limitless You.'" After the first week, Shannon asked Jen if she'd noticed any improvement.

"Well, I guess my speech has improved," Jen said. What an understatement! My daughter had added voice inflections to her speech. You could hear emotions, her speech was much clearer, her movements were better, and her thought process was noticeably quicker. Yes, she had definitely improved. After two weeks of treatment, everyone who came into contact with Jennifer could see the improvement. We had grown accustomed to progressing "inch by inch by inch," but with Brain State Technology the improvement came in a huge leap forward. Even when Jen got back to California her friends commented on the changes.

Twenty years after I first lay on the floor with Emilie Conrad, I realized it might be hugely beneficial to combine Continuum Movement with strength training in a gym. It's hard to believe, but Continuum builds strength itself through its incredibly slow and controlled movements. In particular, it strengthens soft tissue, and it has proven to be beneficial to opening up the tissue before doing anything like weight training. You activate the fluidity of your body and the fluids soften your more linear movements, which is so much better for you.

Once when I came back to California from the East Coast, I asked my neighbor, Paul Adent, a personal trainer, if he'd be willing to work with me. We've been neighbors for over ten years, but until recently, I never felt I was ready for that kind of strain. I had this idea that combining Continuum Movement with strength training in the gym might help my balance. He agreed.

Paul was excited by my request because he knew it would be a challenge for him. He knew where I had come from, and has always been amazed at the progress I've made over the years. The thought of a new avenue towards my recovery—a new blue ribbon to win—was thrilling for me.

Embarrassingly, Paul told me that over the years, he and his partner Paul (we call them "the Pauls") would watch me as I left their apartment, zigzagging down the exterior hallway. The distance from their door to mine was only about fifty feet.

"Do you think she'll make it okay?" Paul would say, and Paul would reply, "I hope so!"

Only recently Paul said to me, "Look at you! That seems like a lifetime ago. I'm so amazed at how far you have come."

And there I was, on a cool spring day, curled up on his couch, drinking chai tea. I couldn't believe that I was about to embark on a new journey and would be able to begin a regime. I started with my Continuum breathing and movement to prepare my body to work with him.

Now I go to the gym twice a week for balance exercises and strength training. Paul also incorporates coordination into my workout, which is good for both my body and my brain. Paul's balance and coordination exercises are challenging, and I have to concentrate just to stay upright. He says, "It is so cool working with you and seeing all your muscles come into play through your determination and focus!" Adding personal training to my weekly routine has awakened even more new pathways in my brain. And I still do Continuum every morning.

Paul Adent, neighbor and personal trainer

Jen moved into our building about ten years ago. I remember wondering at first what caused the pronounced stagger and stumble as she walked down the hallway, swaying dramatically right to left. Was she a bit tipsy? Was she a bit ditsy? What caused the blank stares and delayed responses during conversation? Was she really shy? Why wouldn't she look me directly in the eye?

I also remember she was very kind, funny, and accessible—which were qualities that got her welcomed immediately into our little enclave of neighbors and close friends. Now after more than ten years of really getting to know the ins and outs of Jen—her life, her struggles, her accomplishments, her challenges, her recovery, her story—I am blessed to share a deep, loving friendship.

As a personal trainer, I have been awestruck seeing Jen attack her challenges head on and come out the victor—sometimes with quick results, but more often through laborious determination and a resolve to accept nothing but success and growth. I now have the pleasure of training Jen in the gym, working on both muscle development and balance skills. I sit in admiration when I watch Jen approach an exercise that, to most, would be easy but that challenges every single sensory skill she has worked endlessly to redevelop: sight/spatial perception, hand–eye coordination, motor skills, imbalanced muscular development due to injury and rehab (just to name a few). Her level of determination and concentration is unbelievable and inspiring—she is such a joy to work with.

Now, as I watch her walk in a straight path down the hallway after a wonderful, fluid conversation over tea, I witness and admire her dedication to healing herself, and am inspired firsthand by all the work she is doing to help motivate others by sharing her incredible journey.

In September 2013, I was invited to the General Reinsurance Corporation in Stamford, Connecticut, to speak at a keynote lunch. David Nour, my speaking mentor, made the connection for me, for which I was very grateful. It was my first corporate speaking engagement and was to be streamed over the internet all around the world. This had been a goal for a long time and, although I was nervous, I had practiced long and hard and knew I was prepared. And, as you know, I like being center stage.

*Once again, as during Jen's riding days, I found myself driving unfamiliar roads in Connecticut, thinking about what our hotel would be like and how I would navigate in the dark to the small Italian restaurant we planned to eat at later. But this time, it was not for a horse show and not for therapy. Today was the culmination of every step taken along the way to Jen's recovery. Today my daughter would deliver her inspirational speech, **A Distant Memory**, to the corporate world. I was as nervous as the time she rode into the ring at Madison Square Garden, but equally as proud.*

During the talk, the speakers malfunctioned and kept squeaking like metal on metal, but Jennifer, with her incredible focus, never missed a beat. She delivered her speech flawlessly and I was so proud of her. All of our hard work had paid off. The audience gave her a standing ovation but I couldn't quite read what their full reaction was. They seemed a little bit subdued as they filed out of the room. While we were at lunch in the cafeteria, however, a woman who had been in the audience came up to the table and told Jennifer how incredibly inspiring her speech had been. When the employees returned to their offices, she told us, some of them gathered around not knowing what to say to each other; they had never heard a speech like that. Then, she said, they all started speaking at once about how the speech had affected them in such a positive way. As we were leaving, another woman came running up to tell Jennifer how moved she was, how uplifting the speech would be for anyone in any walk of life, and how she hoped Jen would return to speak again. For us, it was an endorsement not only of the content of Jennifer's speech, but of her delivery as well. It was another success in Jennifer's long journey.

After all these years of struggling, I have finally come into myself. My recovery is an ongoing process, but it gets easier every day. I love being able to help people through my experiences, and I am committed to my foundation and my public speaking. I do feel, still, like I've been given this extra chance at life for a reason, and I think I've found my reason.

I never dreamt any of this would happen. I thought I was a girl who had everything. I never dreamt I would be that girl who lay in a coma in her hospital bed. I never dreamt I would be the person to have to overcome insurmountable obstacles and gain the strength to find my new life. I never could have imagined any of this.

Ironically, it's human nature not to appreciate something until it's gone, or, in my case, taken away. Simple things like breathing, eating, sleeping, walking, enjoying a cup of great coffee, or sharing laughter with friends and family—these are all fundamental things I've learned not to take for granted.

I believe that angels come into our lives in many forms, even in the guise of tragedies and accidents. We haven't done anything wrong. We're not being punished. Struggle teaches us, opens a path towards a new journey. I don't believe we're given any experiences that we can't handle. We somehow find the strength within. In rising to overcome these difficulties, our lives become more enriched, and we grow.

On that cold, snowy November day in 1992, I was given a second chance at life. I began a journey that would reshape my body, my mind, and my spirit. I worked harder than I ever could have imagined. Today I have grown into a person that I love. When I look back, I do not know or recognize the person that I was. I am so different and I have been so humbled. My heart is so much more open, and I have so much more to give. I have been given this second chance at life, and I am determined to honor this incredible gift.

Joanne's Epilogue

The first night of Jennifer's accident, I realized almost immediately that I had to draw from a place inside myself that I never knew existed. I felt like I was balancing on a tightrope and had to keep myself from falling or I would break into a thousand pieces. The idea that Jennifer might be taken from me was so unimaginable that I forced myself to completely shut it out. I prayed, and prayed, and prayed again. At night, while I tried to fall asleep in the day surgery room, I would go to that place inside myself and try to train my brain not to think of the "if onlys" or the "what ifs." I put my brain in a mental cage and told it not to go there. It was too painful. Every once in a while, however, I would succumb, let my thoughts go, and completely break down sobbing.

I was always surrounded by the people whom I loved and who loved Jennifer, but I felt separate. I had to be the one who was strong enough and present enough to make decisions. On that first night in the ICU, people arrived with bottles of wine to begin waiting but I decided I should not drink. I have not taken a drink since.

On that first night in the hospital, a woman called me and told me that her daughter had been in an accident with a horse and had suffered a severe head injury. She told me, above all else, "Stay with your daughter! Don't listen to the doctors! She will get better!" That was a great gift she gave me, and I clung to her advice. It became very clear what my position would be—the person who never left Jen's side, who guarded her, who did everything I could to bring her back. I had no idea what I was getting into, and no idea what the future held, but I honestly believed that if I gave my whole self over to Jennifer's recovery, that maybe I could help reshape her future.

The waiting, the uncertainties, the crises, and the devastating effects of the accident on Jen's body were almost too much to bear. I fought so hard not to break into those thousand pieces. And then, just when I thought I couldn't stand it, she started to come back—an opened eye, an index finger that moved, a whispered "yes," a first mouthful of real food. Those moments were some of the greatest in my life.

When Jennifer was a child she did not talk until she was three. Then one day she ran into the house and said, "Boy, Mom, jumping on the trampoline is so much fun!" I nearly passed out. But when she uttered her first words at age seventeen, in a small halting whisper, I thought I was going to explode with excitement. My mother and I practically danced around the room.

Jennifer's recovery was agonizingly slow, slower than I could ever have imagined, but somehow I knew that we could do it. I always pictured her well, and although it was daunting at times, I always knew that she would recover—in my mind she had to. I turned my whole life over to finding the therapies that I felt would help fix her broken brain and, in turn, her broken body. When I look back I can't believe how many places we went, how many therapies we did—and the incredible excitement I felt when we began to see tiny steps forward. Every day we worked with Jennifer, whether at home or at a new therapy. She worked so hard every day. I can't imagine how it must have been for her as she got better and began to realize all that she had lost, and how much farther she had to go to get better. When I would sense that she was falling into a depression, I would scramble to find a new therapy to get us going again. We never stopped; I felt that if we stopped she might miss a moment when she could have been doing something to make herself better. I was driven and I knew we had to keep going no matter what. Her recovery was the entire focus of my life.

As Jennifer finally made real progress, in the second and third years of her recovery, I could finally picture a real future for her. The day I ran to the barn in my bathrobe, waving her acceptance letter from Wheaton College above my head, I knew we had all climbed to the top of the mountain and that my daughter was going to have a life on her own. How did we come this far? I do believe there were higher powers watching over us. I believe in many ways, I was guided. I believe that I may have been put on this earth to help give my daughter her life back. What greater accomplishment could I achieve than that?

Today, twenty-three years later, when I look at Jennifer delivering her keynote speech and I watch the audience enraptured by her story, my mind travels back as if viewing snapshots of her journey, of the incredibly hard work, and of the courage that brought her to where she is today. I am so proud to have been part of that journey. I am so thankful to have had the help that I had—and I am so grateful that I was able to find the strength to do it.

Jennifer's Epilogue

I THOUGHT MY STORY ENDED WITH DAVID, when I had come full-circle back to a childhood friend after years of struggle. In fact that was *not* the end of the story but only a stop along the way, an important one that I learned from and grew from. David and I parted . . . and I had to travel further to find what I now have today—an incredible man standing by my side and a feeling of fullness and completeness I never knew was possible.

Bruce Dionne entered my life during a casual dog walk. It only took an afternoon for me to be drawn to him by his honesty and generosity. What I have learned from my experiences, my accomplishments, my family, friends, therapists, doctors, other recovering people, and even my audience members, also drew him to me. If I had not been working hard for many years on my health, career, passions, and philanthropy, I never would have noticed Bruce, and he might not have seen me either. Our relationship is a manifestation of who I am now, built from hard work. It wasn't a coincidence that we met; I believe it was meant to be. Our encounter seems an extension of the life that I'd been creating, and that makes being together seem so right.

It started at Burlingame State Park in Rhode Island. I was in nearby Stonington, Connecticut, to work with Molly Ingram on my foundation's newsletter, fundraising projects, and new workshops. She's involved with a dog adoption event group, AlwaysAdopt.com, and she has two whippet rescues, Parker and Peanut, who naturally love to run. At the state park, we joined eight or nine friends with ten or fifteen dogs running free. I remember feeling very precarious in my balance, there on the shore of Watchaug Pond while four huge golden retrievers played wildly close by. Nervous about being bumped or knocked over, I tentatively moved in a small circle, not noticing a friend of Molly's, who she introduced as Bruce. A contractor and carpenter, Bruce worked with AlwaysAdopt.com to help set up the dog adoption days.

From that moment, we just kept walking and talking. He held one of his rescue dogs, Winston, in his arms, and Willie, his other dog, walked closely beside him. Bruce never left my side. I knew the park closed at three o'clock, but we'd arrived at noon and I thought we had plenty of time. The next thing I knew, rangers drove by to tell us it was closing time. Time had flown as we talked; I told him about my accident and recovery, as he told me about his business. I often think twice about talking about all I have been through, but I felt some spark between us. I thought if I told him about my head injury and recovery journey, either he would be standing next to me at the end of the walk or he wouldn't.

When we left the park, we all decided to meet at Galapagos, a coffee bar that sells what I thought was the best coffee I'd had in ages! Or maybe it was the company? My presentation at the LaGrua Center in Stonington was only two days away, so I invited everyone to come hear me speak.

As we were leaving, Molly backed into a wooden gazebo that she claims just magically appeared. When Bruce saw that, he came right over, looked at it, and said he could fix it—a huge relief to Molly. He said he would come back with some wood. "*Wow,*" I thought, "*what a nice guy!*"

Two days later, I stood in front of the crowd at the LaGrua Center, about to deliver *A Distant Memory.* Bruce was there and had brought his mother, Joyce Dionne, which I found touching. They arrived a bit late, and I got nervous pangs that he might not come. But he walked in the door just as I was texting him. His mother, Joyce, had also suffered a head injury, falling downstairs. She related to so much of my talk. Bruce told me that he loved watching her face as she took in what I was saying, nodding her head in agreement. When I looked out into the audience, I was comforted by Bruce's warm, gentle expression.

After my speech, the audience gave me a standing ovation and began crowding around me. I kept Bruce in sight. At last I asked him and his mother to join Molly and me for dinner. Bruce said that his mother was tired, so he would take her home first. The only stipulation I had for dinner was sweet potato fries (I am obsessed with them!). One of our dinner topics was, of all things, Hallmark TV movies. I am so addicted to Hallmark movies that I had even asked Molly if she got the Hallmark Channel. As it turns out, Molly and I are both "happy endings" fans. A new Hallmark movie was on that night; Molly agreed to let Bruce come over and watch it. Her only stipulation, because she was tired, was that he had to drive me home. We shared our first kiss during that movie.

Bruce and I spent the next two days together. Molly and I worked on my annual fundraising appeal letter and on my November newsletter, but I tried to spend every free minute with Bruce. On my last day, he took me to the train station; enveloped in each other's arms, we said goodbye. Definitely a "Hallmark moment!"

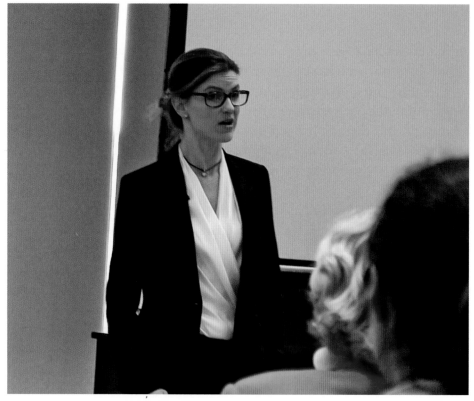

Speaking at the General Reinsurance Corporation 2014

My next speaking engagement was two weeks later in Westbrook, Connecticut, for the Vista Vocational Learning Center. Bruce and I made plans to see each other then, but it felt like an eternity to wait. My mother and I went to Connecticut before my speech to have dinner with my eye doctor, Dr. William Padula, and his wife, Judy. I also had an appointment scheduled with Dr. Padula the next day, when my mom planned to drive to New York for her own appointments. Bruce lived close by in Westerly, Rhode Island, so he agreed to take me to the eye doctor. Afterwards, we had dinner with my mother and friends; everyone liked Bruce.

On the day of my speech, which was also my mother's birthday, Bruce brought his father, Joe Dionne, to see my presentation. "*Wow!*" I thought; I was touched again. It meant so much to see Bruce in the audience.

Just a week later, Bruce came up to Peterborough for the weekend. He fell in love with our historical New England town. I introduced him to family members

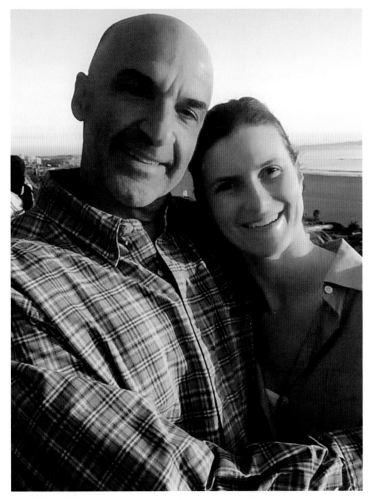

With Bruce

and friends and he was a huge hit. They seemed to see in Bruce all that I saw, which touched me; no difficulty arose to keep Bruce from fitting into my world.

In just a week, I was scheduled to return to California. The day before I left, a friend was driving me from a chiropractor appointment to have a goodbye dinner with my mother. Suddenly, we took a "wrong" turn into a restaurant parking lot. I was just about to say, *"Where are you going?"* when Bruce stepped out of his truck. I couldn't believe I was actually looking into his eyes! He had made the long drive so we could see each other once more before I left. We walked into the restaurant, and

I said, "Look who I found!" We surprised all of them.

I am blessed to be with a kind and generous man. I don't think I have ever known someone able to give so much and always be there. Bruce wants to be everything for me. He has said that I make him feel like more of a man when we are together. I think this is just the beginning of a long, committed relationship. I have learned, over the years, that I crave being in a safe and loving place. I have always been enveloped in a loving home, and have had devoted friends and family, but for some reason I have always felt a part of me was missing. Could it be something my head injury took away? Did it create an emotional hole in me?

Through hard work on my health and career, I have filled many holes during my recovery. Recently, though, people tell me I look more beautiful, taller, and even stronger; perhaps because Bruce is helping me reach a new place of happiness. Like frosting on my cake, I am lucky to have him in my life. Bruce has worked through his own hardships; we connect on many levels.

I do not think a partner is necessary to reach a place of peace and happiness. I was (almost) there on my own. We all can gain happiness and confidence through our own determination and focus. Through my public speaking I knocked on that door and went in. But I have been handed yet another gift—a loving partner who adores me, head injury and all, and wants to travel through life by my side.

Acknowledgments

IT'S BEEN TWENTY-FOUR YEARS since my mother received that horrible phone call from the hospital—the phone call that no parent ever wants to get.

Against all odds, I am here today, and for that I have so many people to thank. Firstly, if not for the late Bill Beynon, the volunteer firefighter who rushed to my mangled car and got me breathing again, I would have died at the scene. Thank you, Bill. You gave me the chance to fight my way back. You were my guardian angel.

From the First Responders, to the Monadnock Community Hospital, to the team at Concord Hospital: I am forever grateful to all the nurses and doctors who worked with my broken body and my damaged brain, step by step, helping me begin to move forward. Thank you to Dr. Albert Butler, the neurosurgeon who flew to Concord from Chicago with my uncle and aunt the night of my accident. Thank you, Angie Dennis, RN, for bending the rules at Concord Hospital so that loving family and friends could surround my mother and me. You knew their presence would be part of my recovery.

Until you are faced with a terrifying situation, you cannot truly know how you will respond. Luckily for me, my mother went into warrior mode. She was determined to get me well, and never took no for an answer. She is the reason I am here today. Mom was then, and remains today, My Champion. And I will always be extremely thankful to my grandmother, who moved heaven and earth to be by my side. She provided strength and direction for my mother.

My mother was not afraid to ask for help. And we got help from so many. That first night Gail Jones, whose daughter had also suffered a terrible head injury, called my mother and told her that I would get better. She also said, "Don't listen to the doctor's prognosis and never leave your daughter's side!" That call provided my mother with a foundation to stand on and the grain of hope she needed to go forward.

Within twenty-four hours after the accident, friends and family began arriving from around the country. My family took over the Concord Hospital ICU waiting room. For the three months I was in a coma, I was never alone. Thank you to all who rallied around my mother and me, providing strength, hope, and even levity. I will be forever grateful to Matt Perlman for giving up months of his life to remain by my side. He was a rock for my mother, and his great sense of humor helped to keep everyone, especially my mom, laughing. Thank you to my friend at the Dublin School, Laura Tolman, who luckily was not in the car with me. Thank you to my cousin Wendy, who was always by our side. And thank you to my friend since I was three, Kristin. She and her mom Carol were always with me. Thank you to Judy Gonzalez for all of her help.

Thank you to my father Edward and his wife Monina, to Bitsy and Sam, for bringing Thanksgiving dinner to the hospital, and always standing by me. Thank you John "The Crisis Buster" and his wife Peggy. Thank you to Uncle Marsh and Aunt Jamee, with whom my mother and I stayed for several months when I went to Chicago for more therapy. I could never possibly thank them enough for everything they did for me!

Our dear friend and property caretaker, Michael Martin, stuck by us through it all and eventually became my physical therapist, helping me with my exercises and treatments. Mike was the keystone of my recovery team, working with me every day from dawn until dusk, and taking me to appointments near and far. He provided strength and a sense of sanity for both my mother and me.

Thank you to Dr. James Whitlock and Northeast Rehabilitation for providing me with top rehabilitation.

Thank you to the Rehabilitation Institute of Chicago and to the late Dr. Henry Betts who looked over me when I was in Chicago.

Thank you Dr. William Padula for providing exceptional vision therapy, and for his ever-thoughtful advice.

Thank you Dr. Patricia Kane, Alice Quaid, and Jacques Marin for giving me back a piece of myself.

Thank you to my nutritionist and friend Dr. Tobin Watkinson.

I would like to honor and give thanks to some of the most important people in my recovery who are no longer with us: Emilie Conrad, Founder of Continuum, who became the light at the end of my tunnel; Dr. Bernard Brucker, who gave me back a heel strike and so much more; Dr. Upledger, who was a master of craniosacral manipulation; Dr. Christine Nelson in Cuernavaca, Mexico, who was a physical therapy genius; Margaret Ayers, another genius and an early pioneer in the field of neurofeedback; and Martha Estin, who set me on my road back with her cross patterning. These people were my angels. They each saw me as a person as well as a patient, and found ways to work with me that opened doors and windows to me. They rejected current thinking and dared to believe my brain and my body could heal.

Thank you to the Dublin School for allowing me to graduate with my class. Thank you to Wheaton College for taking a chance on me when I decided I wanted to get my college degree. Thank you to Evelyn Staudinger and Pozzi Escot for making my experience at Wheaton so special.

Thank you to Alan Weiss, David Nour, and Lou Heckler for believing in my dream as much as I did. Your guidance helped me achieve my goal of being an inspirational keynote speaker.

Thank you to Grove Street Books for sticking with us and for publishing *From Blue Ribbon to Code Blue*.

And finally, I want to give special thanks to my friend Sue Scott, without whom this book would not have been possible. Sue, who cheered me on throughout my recovery, spent endless hours with my mother and me, helping us to pull out deeply buried memories and anecdotes to tell our story.